INTRODUCTION

So, you've decided to change your life! Congratulations! I'm Evelyn Leigh and I designed this journal to cater to all my needs during my health and wellness journey, Then I realized how helpful it would be to share this with you all. The Sleigh By Leigh Journey Tracker is a 12 month undated planner dedicated to aligning your physical, mental and spiritual health in order to have a successful fitness journey. Undated because hiccups are inevitable and should you happen to have one yourself, you can just pick right up like nothing ever happened! This journal is designed for you to be completely honest with yourself and hold yourself accountable. Whether you are looking to lose or gain weight, this journal will certainly help you map out a plan and stick to it! With self care reminders, gratitude logs, sleep trackers, meal planners and more, you are bound to reach ALL your goals and "SLEIGH" this journey! Wishing you the best of luck and if you ever need some advice, tips, recipes or motivation, follow @SleighByLeigh! I'm on this journey with you and am more than happy to help!

MANTRA

A personal mantra is an affirmation used to motivate and inspire you to be your best self. A mantra provides the motivation and encouragement you need to focus your mind on achieving a goal. Originating in Buddhism and Hinduism, mantras were words or sounds that aided in concentration during meditation. Here you will use this portion to write your very own mantra with a personal goal, being overall health and happiness. It can be as long or short as you'd like, but remember, you will start each day repeating this to yourself and eventually will memorize it. Use positive words such as "I will", "When I", I can", I am", etc. Speak all you want to achieve on this journey and beyond into existence. A main component in these exercises is to encourage positive thinking and speaking over yourself. Don't overthink. Just express freely.

WEIGH IN

Here is where you'll list your weigh ins. Each round consists of one month and you will weigh in weekly. It's best to decide on a preferred day you'd like to weigh in on. (Ex: Sundays or Wednesdays). Creating a routine will greatly benefit you on this journey. Each weigh in you'll list your current weight and the date in the boxes below. You will also provide your goal weight for that round and list something you plan to reward yourself with when you achieve your goal. At the end of the round you will list your final weigh in. If you achieved your goal, reward yourself and even if you haven't, no worries! You are doing your absolute best and will achieve that goal!

ROUND 1

GOAL: REWARD: FINAL:

ROUND 2

GOAL: REWARD: FINAL:

ROUND 3

GOAL: REWARD: FINAL:

ROUND 4

GOAL: REWARD: FINAL:

WEIGH IN

ROUND 5

GOAL: REWARD: FINAL:

ROUND 6

GOAL: REWARD: FINAL:

ROUND 7

GOAL: REWARD: FINAL:

ROUND 8

GOAL: REWARD: FINAL:

WEIGH IN

ROUND
9

GOAL: REWARD: FINAL:

ROUND
10

GOAL: REWARD: FINAL:

ROUND
11

GOAL: REWARD: FINAL:

ROUND
12

GOAL: REWARD: FINAL:

MEASUREMENT TRACKER

Here is where you'll track your measurements. Each round you will measure all listed areas of your body and jot them down here. Unlike the weigh in goals, which are monthly, you'll set a measurement goal for yourself every 3 months. This will give you ample time to achieve your goal and drop a size or two. Also a good thing to remember, if you're not losing as much as you expect, it's always possible that you are losing inches, which is just as great! List a reward for when you achieve your measurement goals. The goal incentive encourages you to treat yourself in a way you might not usually while also making sure that you're celebrating EVERY accomplishment you make.

	CHEST	WAIST	HIPS	L ARM	R ARM	L THIGH	R THIGH
JAN							
FEB							
MAR							
APR							
MAY							
JUN							
JUL							
AUG							
SEP							
OCT							
NOV							
DEC							

ROUND 3 GOALS

ROUND 6 GOALS

ROUND 9 GOALS

ROUND 12 GOALS

ROUND 1

And so, the journey begins.

Difficult roads often lead to beautiful destinations. The best is *yet* to come.
Zig Ziglar

GOALS

Each round consists of one month. List a few of your goals for this round here. Be honest and don't overwhelm yourself. You have 4 weeks to achieve these goals. Include fitness goals, habits you'd like to break and self care as well. Have fun!

GETTING TO KNOW YOU

This portion is for you to get to know yourself a little better before we start the first round of your journey. You will do these every 3 rounds. It's a reflection that you'll be happy to look back on at the end of your yearlong journey. Write a short letter to yourself explaining who you are at this point in your life and what has inspired you to embark on this journey. Be honest with yourself. No one will read this but you. Don't overthink it. Just write freely.

HABIT TRACKER

Here is where you'll track your habits in the boxes below. Number the boxes accordingly for the month you're in and jot down the name of the habit you are working towards or determined to break. (Ex: Fast food, Exercise, Smoking, etc.) Each day you are successful in either achieving or breaking this habit, you'll color in the box on that date. The ultimate goal as you continue on through your rounds is to have the whole month colored in. The key is to break bad habits and enforce good ones.

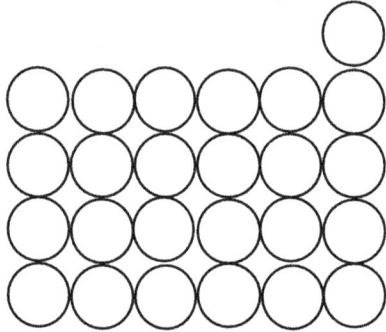

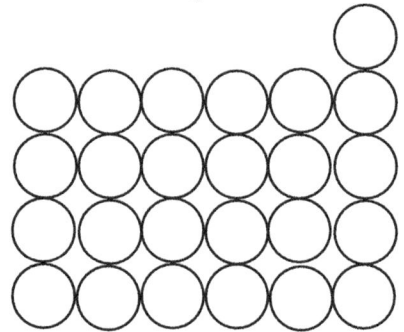

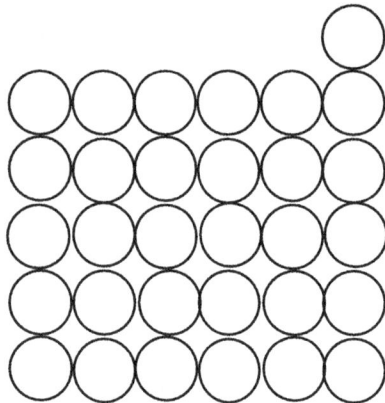

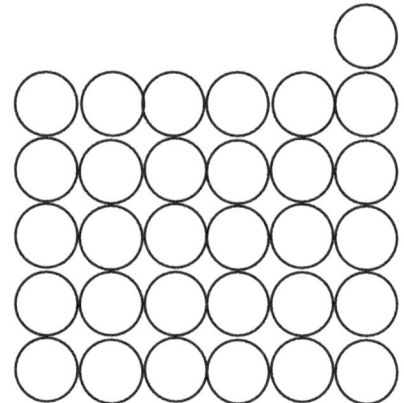

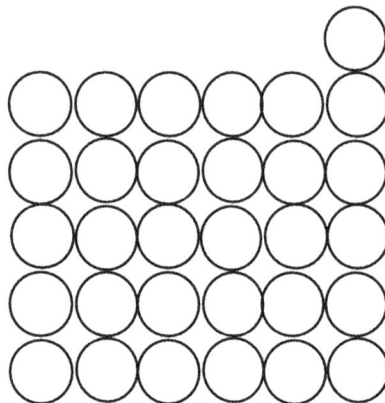

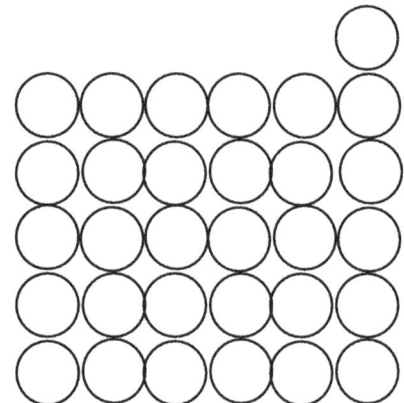

MOOD TRACKER

Here is where you'll track your moods daily. Each round you will do this to track how you're feeling throughout your journey. In the "Key" box below, choose your moods and colors to represent them. Each day color in the hearts according to your mood. You're allowed to have good days and bad days. It's perfectly normal throughout your journey. It's called a journey for a reason, you aren't to be in the same place the entire time. Your health, mental state and appearance are all subject to change. Allow yourself to be human and allow yourself the necessary room to grow.

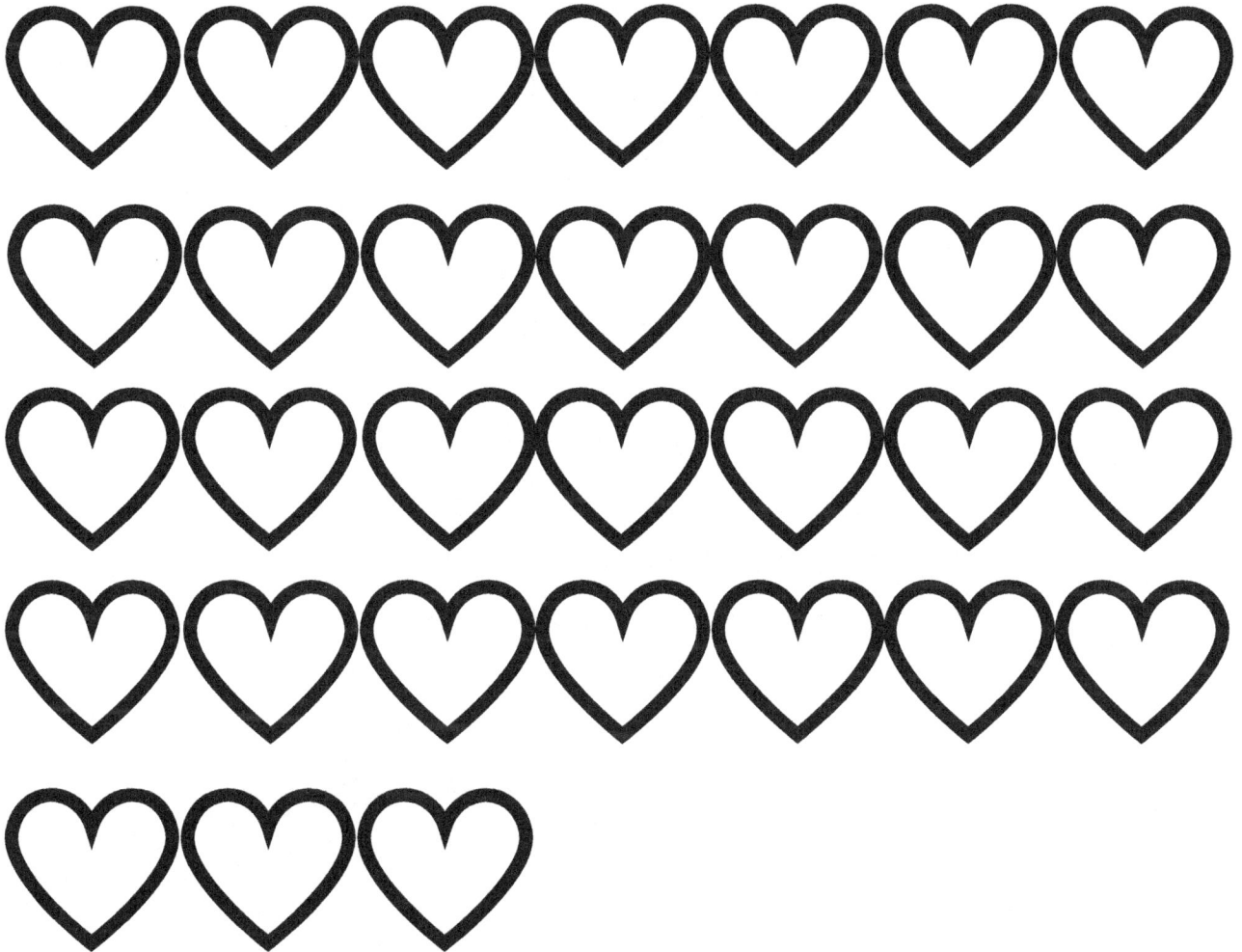

KEY:

Self Care Reminder

Fill this page up with your ideas of self care. When you've completed that task, highlight it. Include everything that caters to your mind, body and soul. Self care is more than face masks and bubble baths. Trusting yourself + doing what is in your best interest is self care.

MENTAL HEALTH CHECK IN

This portion is a free write. Come back here as often as you'd like to pour out your feelings of how your journey is going. Some days are much harder than others and its helpful to get it out your head and jot it down. Just a few minutes a day, take a moment to free your mind here. You'll like to look back on this as well throughout your journey to reflect on your mindset at the start of your journey.

GRATITUDE LOG

This portion is a free write. Come back here as often as you'd like to pour out your feelings of gratitude during this round. You'll like to look back on this as well throughout your journey to reflect on your mindset at the start of your journey.

MONTH OVERVIEW

This undated calendar is for you to track and schedule activities.
Anything from work to preferred gym days, meal planning, and even mental
health days. Use the "Key" box below to color code all your plans and activities.
Think of it as a "YOU" calender. Everything YOU need to do for yourself to be
successful on this journey, plan it all out here.

S	M	T	W	T	F	S

KEY

MEAL PLANNING

This portion is for planning meals ahead. Come back here as often as you'd like
to plan your meals or even make grocery lists. You'll like to look back on this as well
throughout your journey to reflect on your mindset at the start of your journey.

	S	M	T	W
BREAKFAST				
LUNCH				
DINNER				
SNACKS				

MEAL PLANNING

T	F	S	SHOPPING LIST

WORKOUT LOG

This portion is for logging all physical activity. Gym, walks, yoga, zumba, etc. Even sexy time.Yes, the club counts. If you sweat, it counts. Use the "Key" box below to color code all your activities. This is a no pressure portion. If you rested, write "rest day". If you didn't exercise at all, write "N/A". The ultimate goal is to be as active as often possible and create a healthy habit of physical activity.

	S	M	T	W	T	F	S
WEEK 1							
WEEK 2							
WEEK 3							
WEEK 4							

KEY

SLEEP TRACKER

31
30
29
28
27
26
25
24
23
22
21
20
19
18
17
16
15
14
13
12
11
10
9
8
7
6
5
4
3
2
1

6 7 8 9 10 11 12 1 2 3 4 5 6 7 8 9 10 11 12

This portion is for tracking the amount of sleep you're getting regularly. Tracking your sleep pattern will help you determine what to implement in your routine for a good night's sleep. Each day place a dot on the hour you fell asleep and place another on the hour you woke up. Then connect those dots.

Name 5 things you accomplished today.

Name 5 things that made you smile.

Name 5 things that worried/frightened/ stressed you.

Name 5 things that you did for yourself today.

Name 5 things you plan to accomplish tomorrow.

Nightly prayer/express gratitude.

Nightly Exercise

Unplug before bed. avoid tv/phone/ etc. read or even journal before bed.

Try a lavender incense or pillow spray.

Take a bubble bath/shower. soak in epsom salts or add a few drops of lavender oil.

Try Celestial's Sleepytime teas.

Find a pleasing sound to fall asleep to on the "Rain Rain" app. Its Free!

Trouble Sleeping?

MEAL TRACKER

This portion is for logging all your meals and water intake daily. Log everything, even the junk food. Use the "Water" box and color in a glass for every glass of water you've consumed that day. Tracking everything you eat is helpful to hold yourself accountable and see what changes need to be made in your weekly meals. For example, if you consumed a lot of sweets this week, then next week you'll focus on cutting down or out sweets completely. Whether or not you've committed to a specific diet, this portion will help you set goals and notice your eating habits. The ultimate goal is to eventually make as many healthy options as possible and replace bad eating habits with better ones.

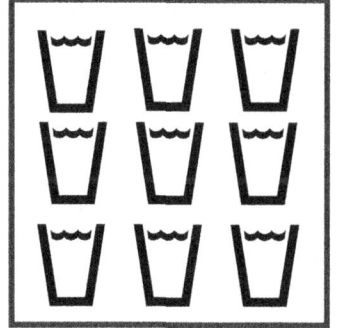

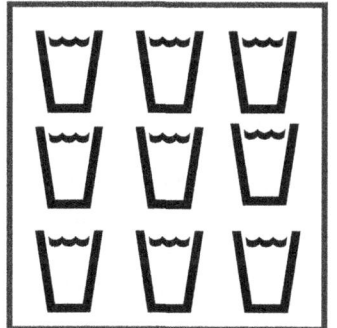

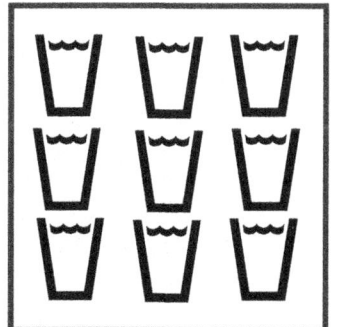

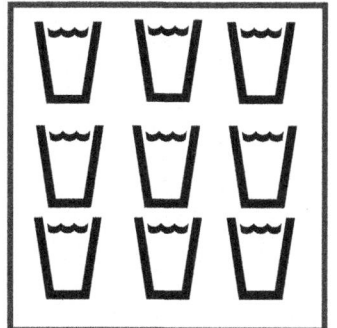

MEAL TRACKER

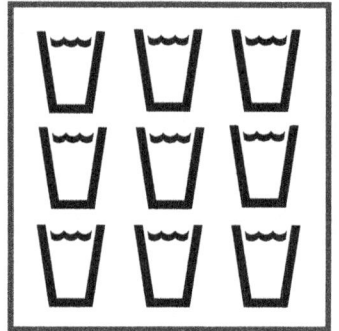

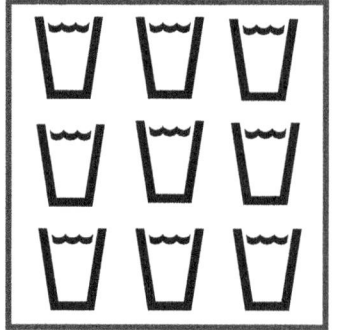

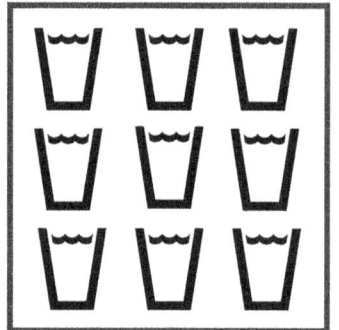

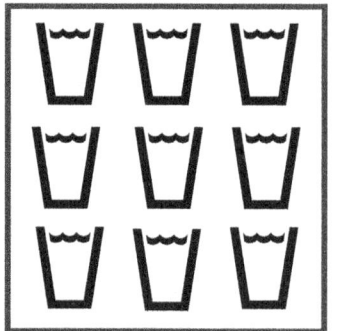

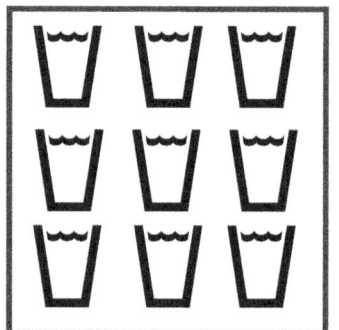

MEAL TRACKER

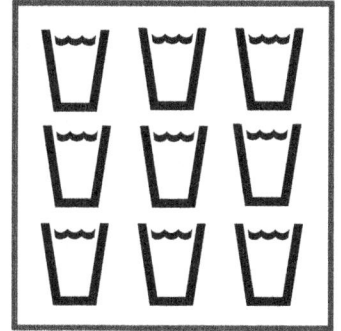

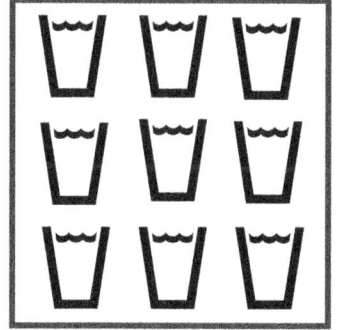

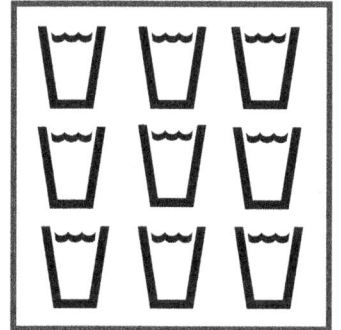

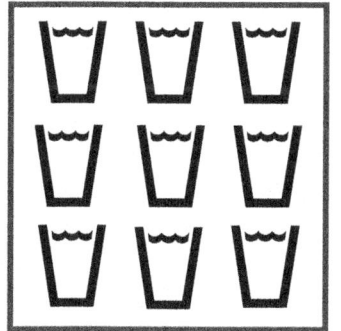

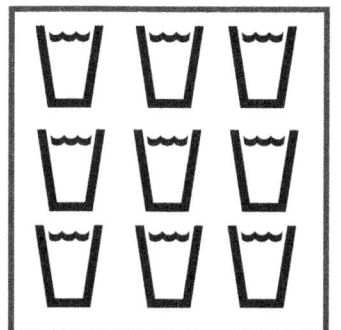

MEAL TRACKER

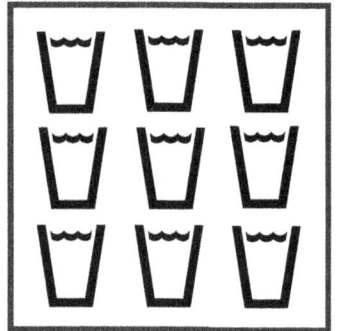

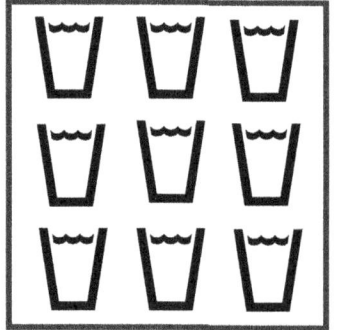

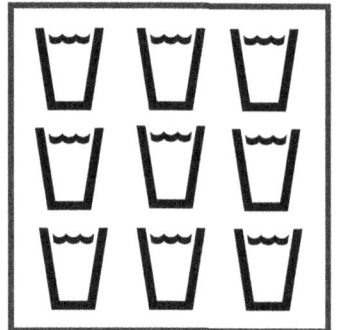

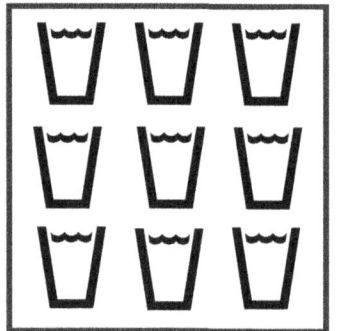

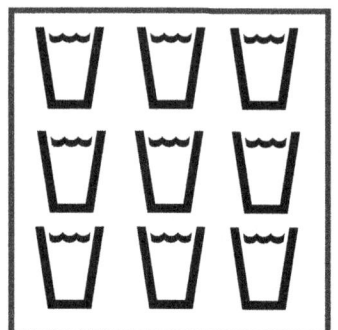

MEAL TRACKER

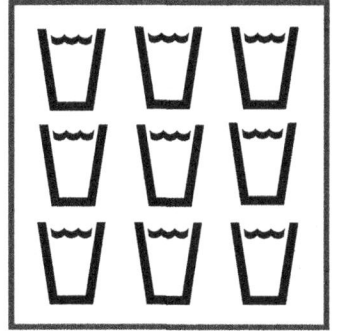

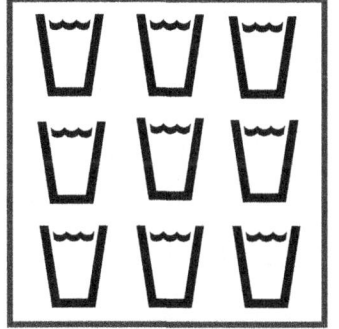

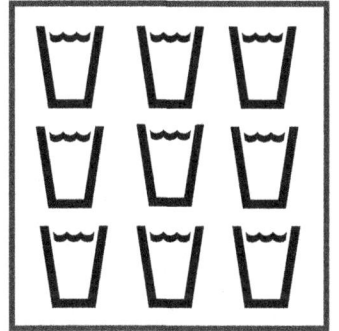

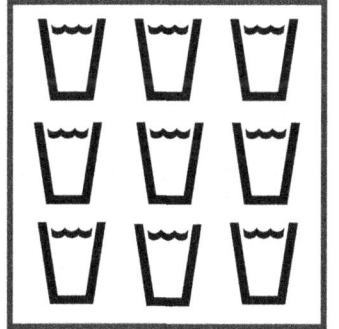

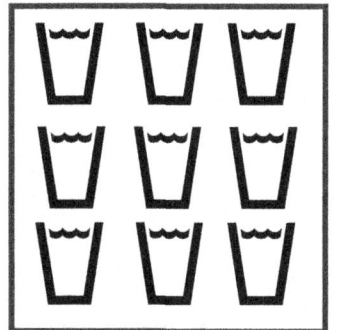

MEAL TRACKER

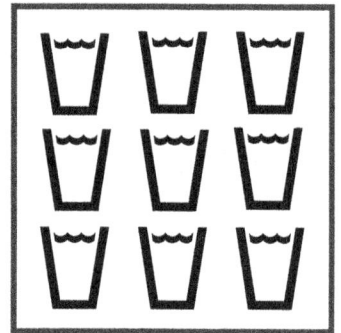

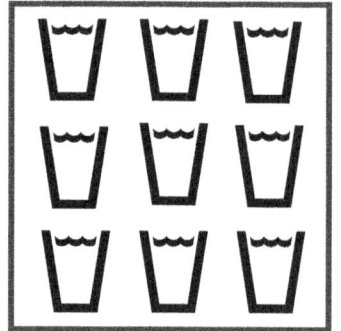

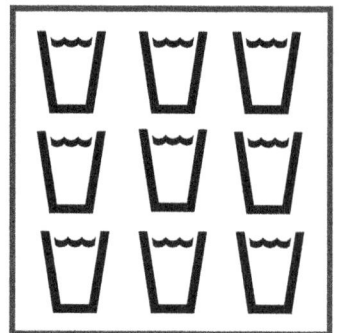

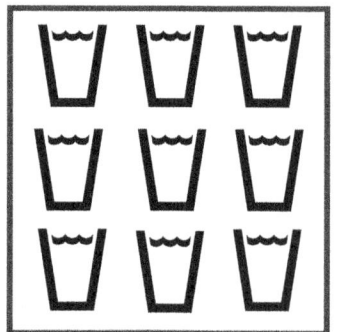

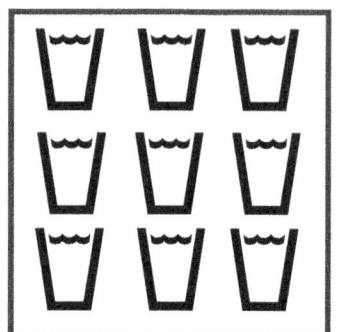

MEAL TRACKER

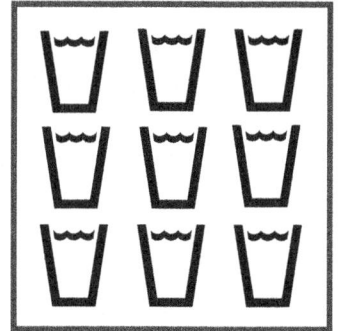

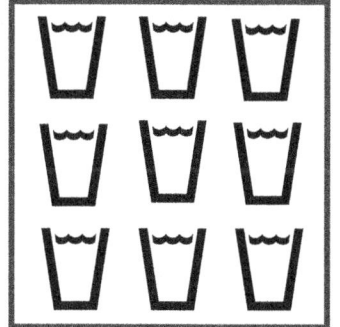

ROUND OVERVIEW

How many times did you eat fast food?

How many times did you cook your own meals?

Did you step out of your comfort zone with any meals?

How was your water intake?

What do you plan to change about your meals next round?

List 3 meals you'd like to cut out.

List 3 new meals you'd like to try.

ROUND OVERVIEW

DID YOU ACCOMPLISH YOUR GOAL WEIGHT? IF YES, WHAT DID YOU REWARD YOURSELF WITH AND WHY?

WERE YOU SUCCESSFUL IN CONTROLLING OR ENDING ANY BAD HABITS? WHICH HABITS DO YOU THINK WILL REQUIRE MORE OF YOUR TIME? DID YOU TAKE ON ANY GOOD HABITS? WHAT WERE THEY? WHAT HABITS ARE YOU INTERESTED IN WORKING ON NEXT ROUND?

HOW WERE YOUR MOODS THIS MONTH? WHAT HAVE YOU DONE FOR YOURSELF? HOW DO YOU FEEL AFTER COMPLETING THIS ROUND?

HOW'D THE SELF CARE REMINDER GO? HOW MANY TIMES DID YOU CATER TO YOURSELF? WHAT DO YOU HAVE PLANNED TO TREAT YOURSELF NEXT ROUND?

DID YOU TRY MEAL PLANNING THIS MONTH? DISCOVER ANY NEW RECIPES OR FOODS YOU ENJOYED? CHOOSE A DAY THAT WOULD BE GOOD FOR YOU TO MEAL PREP FOR THE WEEK.

HOW ACTIVE WERE YOU THIS ROUND? WHAT WAS YOUR MOST FREQUENT ACTIVITY? HOW DO YOU PLAN TO BE MORE ACTIVE NEXT ROUND? ANYTHING NEW YOU'D LIKE TO TRY?

WHAT DID YOUR SLEEP TRACKER REVEAL? HOW HAS IT CHANGED? TRY ANY OF OF THE TIPS/EXERCISES? WHICH ONES WERE HELPFUL?

ROUND 2

GOOD THINGS TAKE TIME.

I can and I will.

WATCH ME.

Unknown

GOALS

Each round consists of one month. List a few of your goals for this round here. Be honest and don't overwhelm yourself. You have 4 weeks to achieve these goals. Include fitness goals, habits you'd like to break and self care as well. Have fun!

HABIT TRACKER

Here is where you'll track your habits. In this round the dates are provided so jot down the name of the habit you are working towards or determined to break on the line below. (Ex: Fast food, Exercise, Smoking, etc.) Each day you are successful in either achieving or breaking this habit, you'll highlight or circle the date. The ultimate goal as you continue on through your rounds is to have the whole month colored in. The key is to break bad habits and enforce good ones.

1 2 3 4 5 6 7 8 9
10 11 12 13 14 15 16
17 18 19 20 21 22 23
24 25 26 27 28 29
30 31

_____

1 2 3 4 5 6 7 8 9
10 11 12 13 14 15 16
17 18 19 20 21 22 23
24 25 26 27 28 29
30 31

_____

1 2 3 4 5 6 7 8 9
10 11 12 13 14 15 16
17 18 19 20 21 22 23
24 25 26 27 28 29
30 31

_____

1 2 3 4 5 6 7 8 9
10 11 12 13 14 15 16
17 18 19 20 21 22 23
24 25 26 27 28 29
30 31

_____

MOOD TRACKER

Here is where you'll track your moods daily. Each round you will do this to track how you're feeling throughout your journey. In the "Key" box below, choose your moods and colors to represent them. Each day color in the hearts according to your mood. You're allowed to have good days and bad days. It's perfectly normal throughout your journey. It's called a journey for a reason, you aren't to be in the same place the entire time. Your health, mental state and appearance are all subject to change. Allow yourself to be human and allow yourself the necessary room to grow.

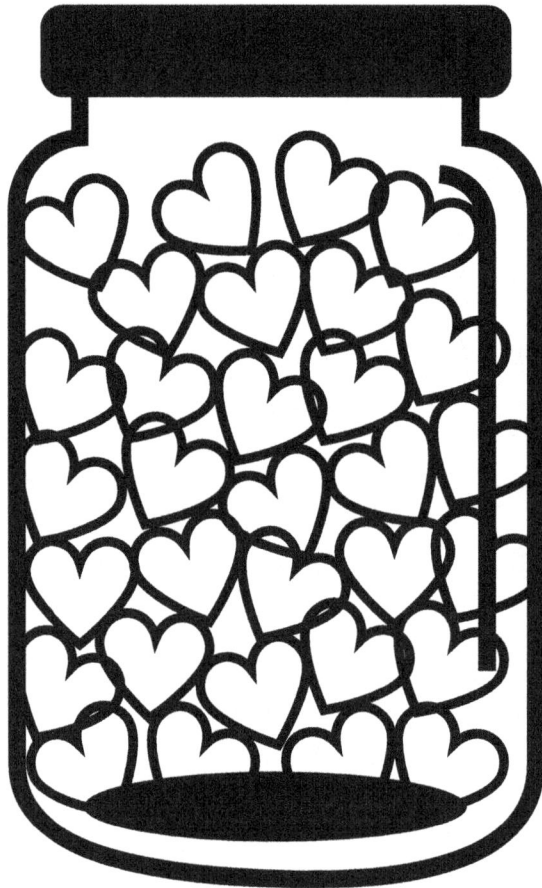

KEY:

ACTS OF SELF CARE

Fill the boxes below with your ideas of self care for your body, mind and soul. When you've completed that task, highlight it or cross it out. Include everything that caters to your mind, body and soul. Self care is more than face masks and bubble baths. Trusting yourself + doing what is in your best interest is self care.

MIND

BODY

SOUL

MENTAL HEALTH CHECK IN

This portion is a free write. Come back here as often as you'd like to pour out your feelings of how your journey is going. Some days are much harder than others and its helpful to get it out your head and jot it down. Just a few minutes a day, take a moment to free your mind here. You'll like to look back on this as well throughout your journey to reflect on your mindset at the start of your journey.

GRATITUDE LOG

This portion is a free write. Come back here as often as you'd like to pour out your feelings of gratitude during this round. You'll like to look back on this as well throughout your journey to reflect on your mindset at the start of your journey.

MONTH OVERVIEW

This undated calendar is for you to track and schedule activities.Anything from work to preferred gym days, meal planning, and even mental health days. Use the "Key" box below to color code all your plans and activities. Think of it as a "YOU" calendar.Everything YOU need to do for yourself to be successful on this journey, plan it all out here.

S	M	T	W	T	F	S

KEY

MEAL PLANNING

This portion is for planning meals ahead. Come back here as often as you'd like to plan your meals or even make grocery lists. You'll like to look back on this as well throughout your journey to reflect on your mindset at the start of your journey.

	S	M	T	W
BREAKFAST				
LUNCH				
DINNER				
SNACKS				

MEAL PLANNING

This portion is for planning meals ahead. Come back here as often as you'd like to plan your meals or even make grocery lists. You'll like to look back on this as well throughout your journey to reflect on your mindset at the start of your journey.

T	F	S	SHOPPING LIST

WORKOUT LOG

	S	M	T	W	T	F	S
WEEK 1							
WEEK 2							
WEEK 3							
WEEK 4							

KEY

SLEEP TRACKER

31
30
29
28
27
26
25
24
23
22
21
20
19
18
17
16
15
14
13
12
11
10
9
8
7
6
5
5
3
2
1

6 7 8 9 10 11 12 1 2 3 4 5 6 7 8 9 10 11 12

MEAL TRACKER

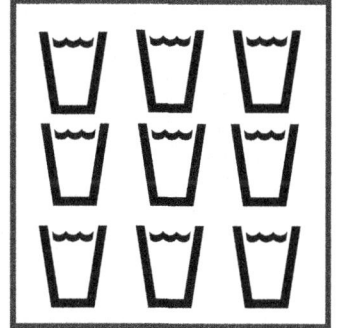

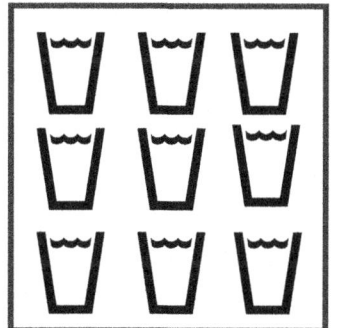

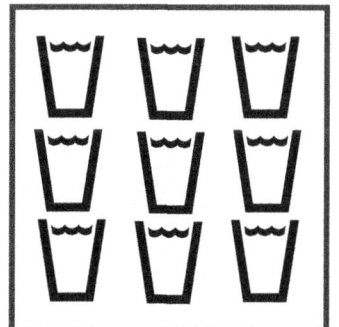

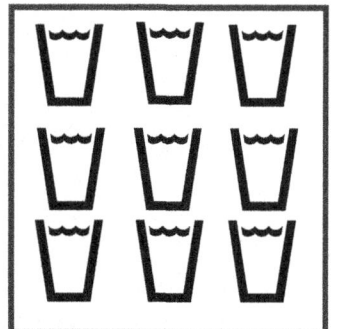

MEAL TRACKER

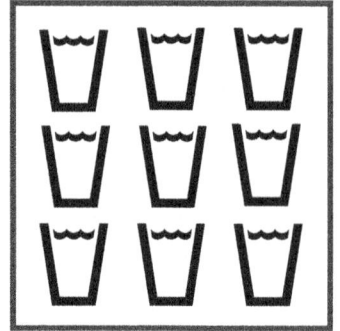

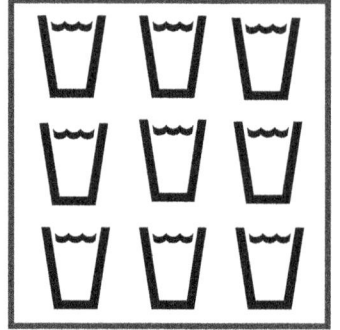

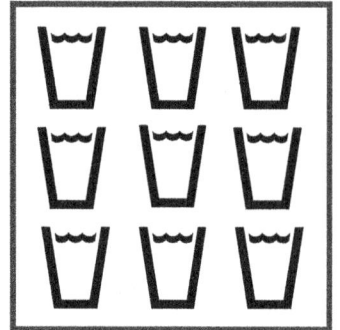

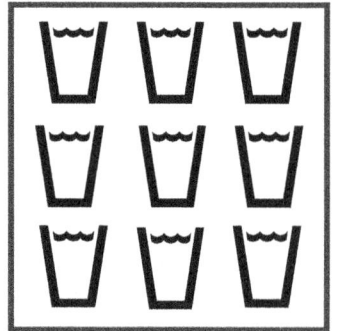

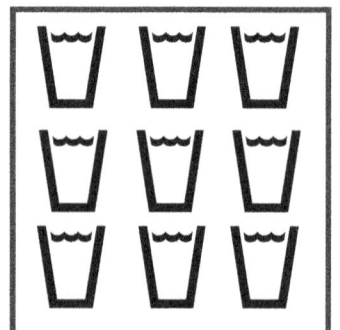

MEAL TRACKER

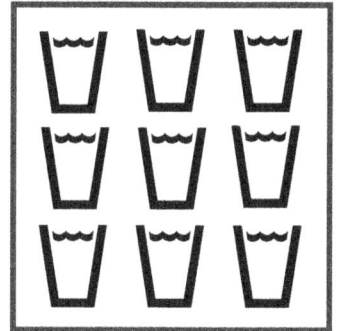

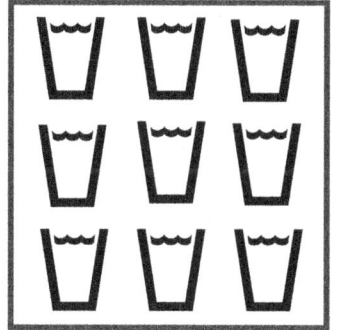

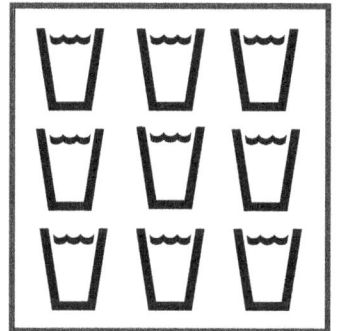

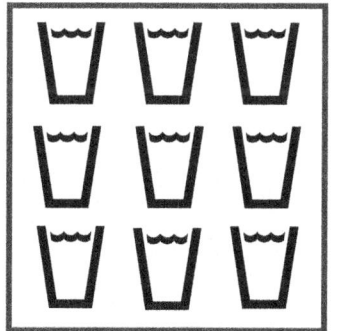

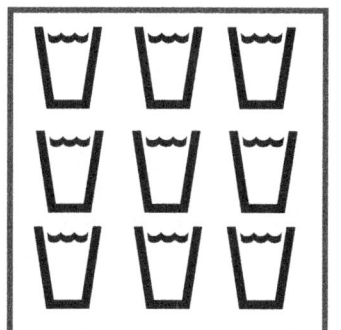

MEAL TRACKER

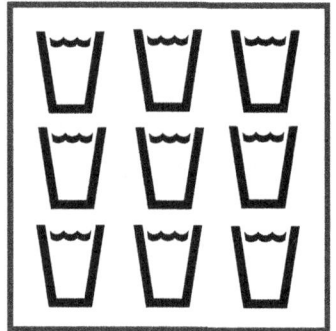

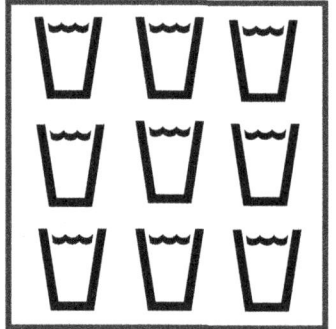

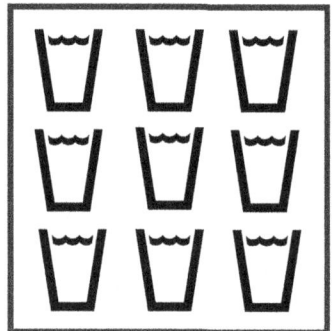

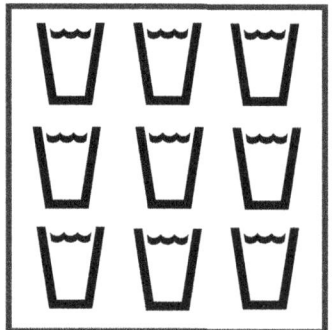

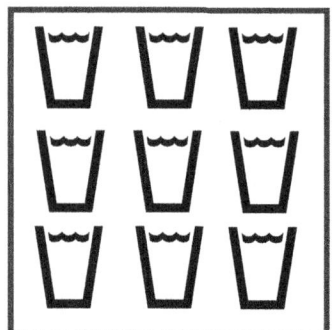

MEAL TRACKER

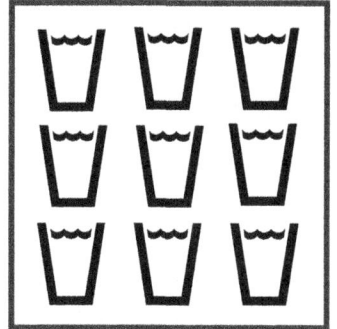

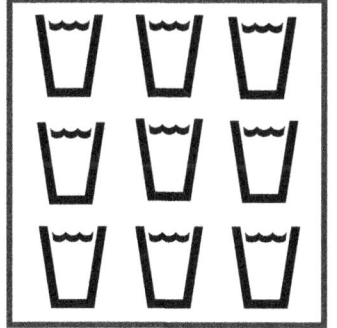

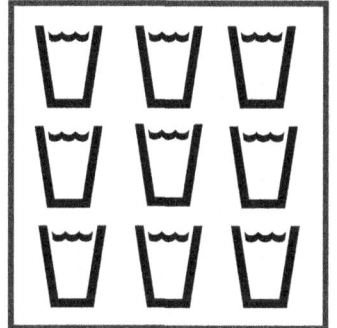

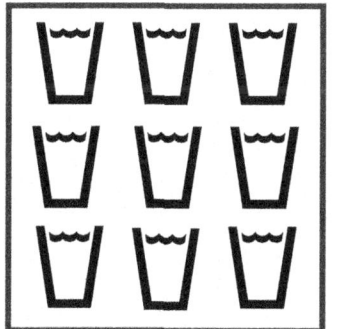

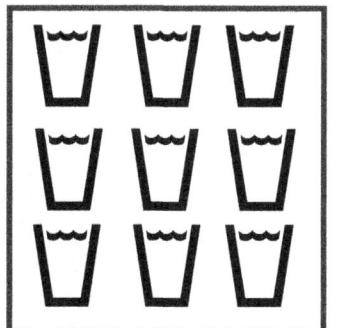

MEAL TRACKER

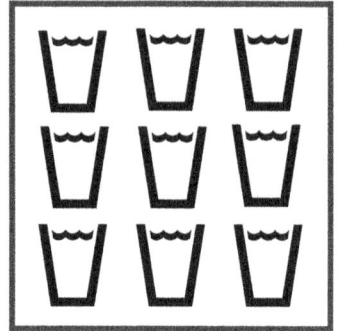

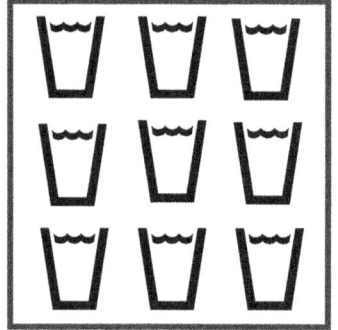

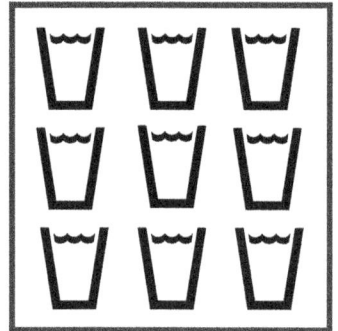

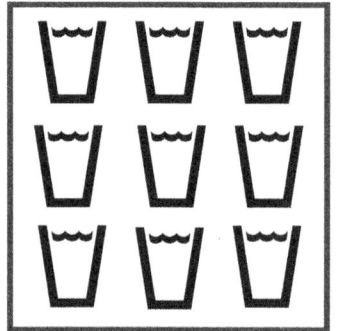

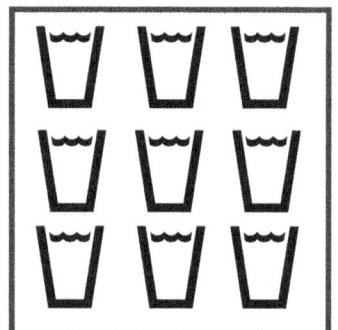

MEAL TRACKER

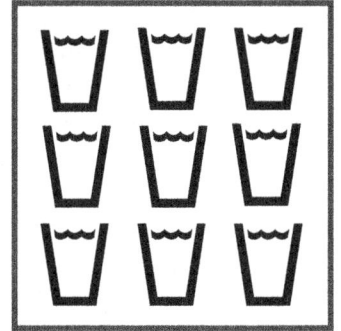

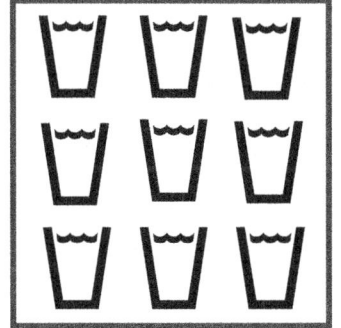

ROUND OVERVIEW

How many times did you eat fast food?

How many times did you cook your own meals?

Did you step out of your comfort zone with any meals?

How was your water intake?

What do you plan to change about your meals next round?

List 3 meals you'd like to cut out.

List 3 new meals you'd like to try.

ROUND OVERVIEW

DID YOU ACCOMPLISH YOUR GOAL WEIGHT? IF YES, WHAT DID YOU REWARD YOURSELF WITH AND WHY?

WERE YOU SUCCESSFUL IN CONTROLLING OR ENDING ANY BAD HABITS? WHICH HABITS DO YOU THINK WILL REQUIRE MORE OF YOUR TIME? DID YOU TAKE ON ANY GOOD HABITS? WHAT WERE THEY? WHAT HABITS ARE YOU INTERESTED IN WORKING ON NEXT ROUND?

HOW WERE YOUR MOODS THIS MONTH? WHAT HAVE YOU DONE FOR YOURSELF? HOW DO YOU FEEL AFTER COMPLETING THIS ROUND?

HOW'D THE SELF CARE REMINDER GO? HOW MANY TIMES DID YOU CATER TO YOURSELF? WHAT DO YOU HAVE PLANNED TO TREAT YOURSELF NEXT ROUND?

DID YOU TRY MEAL PLANNING THIS MONTH? DISCOVER ANY NEW RECIPES OR FOODS YOU ENJOYED? CHOOSE A DAY THAT WOULD BE GOOD FOR YOU TO MEAL PREP FOR THE WEEK.

HOW ACTIVE WERE YOU THIS ROUND? WHAT WAS YOUR MOST FREQUENT ACTIVITY? HOW DO YOU PLAN TO BE MORE ACTIVE NEXT ROUND? ANYTHING NEW YOU'D LIKE TO TRY?

WHAT DID YOUR SLEEP TRACKER REVEAL? HOW HAS IT CHANGED? TRY ANY OF OF THE TIPS/EXERCISES? WHICH ONES WERE HELPFUL?

ROUND 3

FRIENDS + FAMILY   CAREER

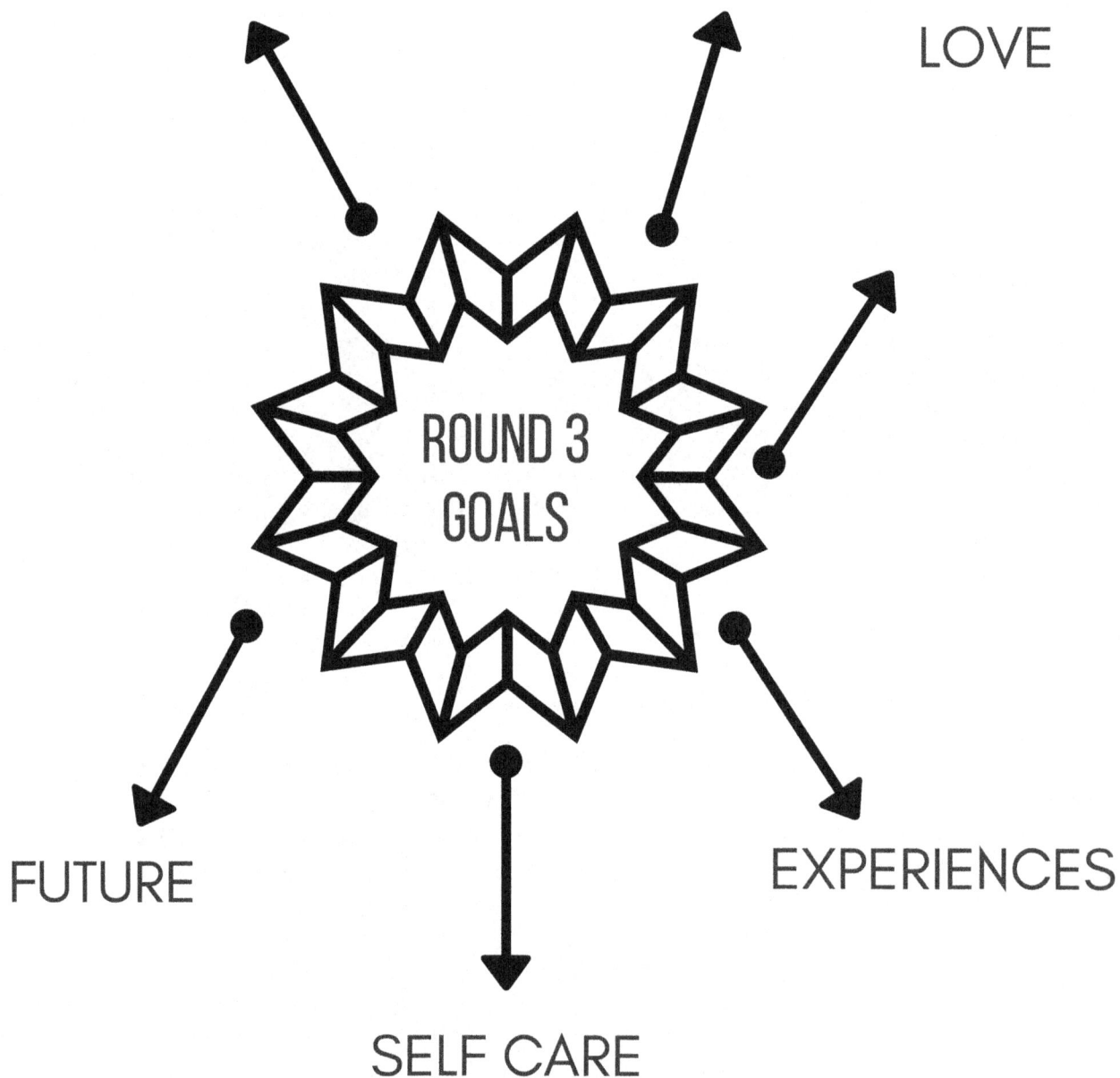

LOVE

ROUND 3
GOALS

FUTURE

EXPERIENCES

SELF CARE

HABIT TRACKER

Here is where you'll track your habits. In this round the dates are provided so jot down the name of the habit you are working towards or determined to break on the line below. (Ex: Fast food, Exercise, Smoking, etc.) Each day you are successful in either achieving or breaking this habit, you'll highlight or circle the date. The ultimate goal as you continue on through your rounds is to have the whole month colored in. The key is to break bad habits and enforce good ones.

1 2 3 4 5 6 7 8 9
10 11 12 13 14 15 16
17 18 19 20 21 22 23
24 25 26 27 28 29
30 31

_____

1 2 3 4 5 6 7 8 9
10 11 12 13 14 15 16
17 18 19 20 21 22 23
24 25 26 27 28 29
30 31

_____

1 2 3 4 5 6 7 8 9
10 11 12 13 14 15 16
17 18 19 20 21 22 23
24 25 26 27 28 29
30 31

_____

1 2 3 4 5 6 7 8 9
10 11 12 13 14 15 16
17 18 19 20 21 22 23
24 25 26 27 28 29
30 31

_____

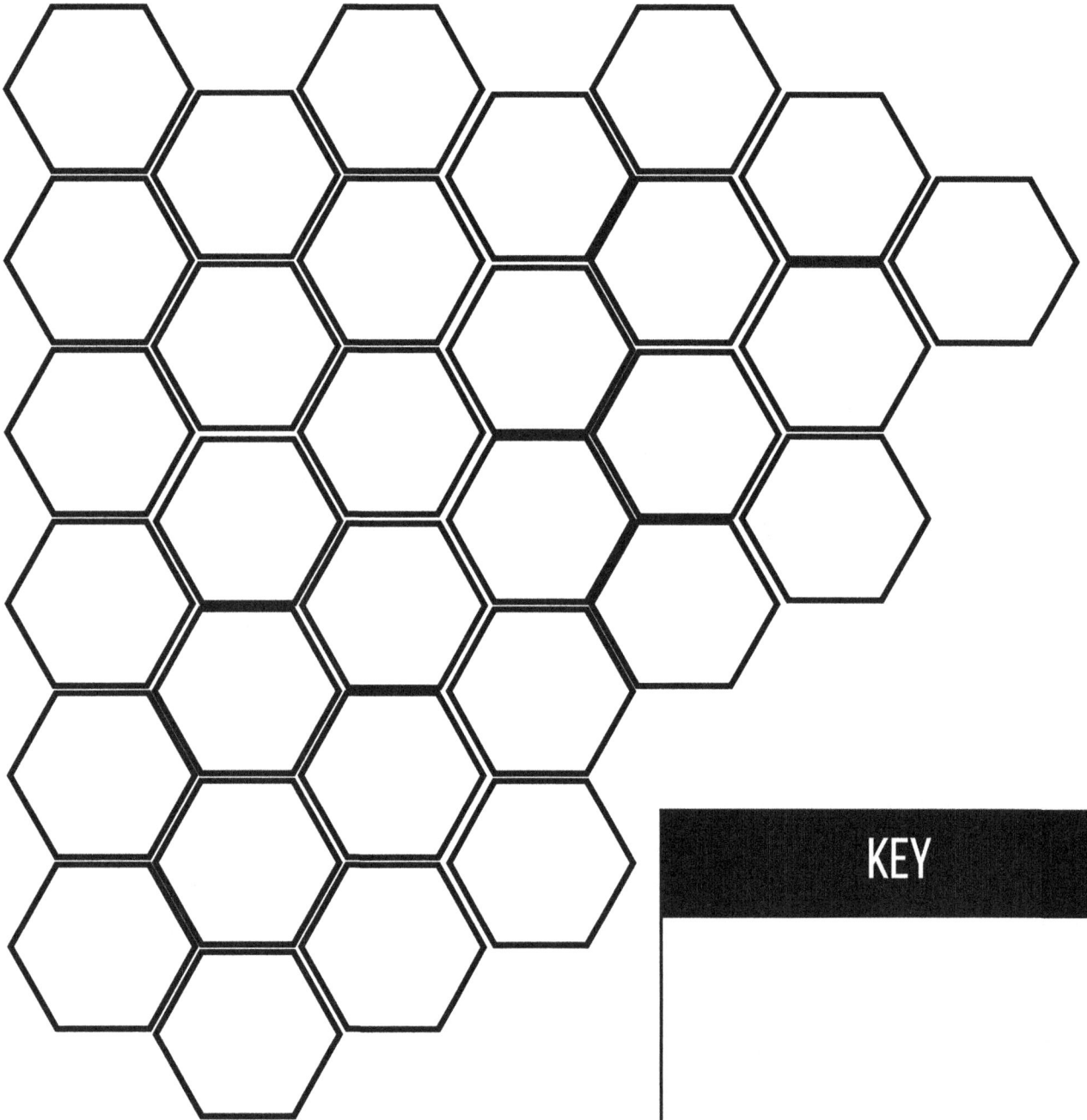

MOOD TRACKER

KEY

What Makes Me Happy?

This portion is a little different than the others. Here you will fill this page with ANY and EVERYTHING that makes you happy. This is a reflecting portion.

30 DAYS OF SELF CARE

For this portion you will list 30 acts of self care for each day this month. This is a challenge for you to spend a bit more time taking care of yourself. Be sure to include physical, mental and spiritual acts for the month. Cater to your overall health. When you've completed that task, come back and highlight it.

S	M	T	W	T	F	S

KEY

MENTAL HEALTH CHECK IN

This portion is a free write. Come back here as often as you'd like to pour out your feelings of how your journey is going. Some days are much harder than others and its helpful to get it out your head and jot it down. Just a few minutes a day, take a moment to free your mind here. You'll like to look back on this as well throughout your journey to reflect on your mindset at the start of your journey.

GRATITUDE LOG

This portion is a free write. Come back here as often as you'd like to pour out your feelings of gratitude during this round. You'll like to look back on this as well throughout your journey to reflect on your mindset at the start of your journey.

MONTH OVERVIEW

This undated calendar is for you to track and schedule activities. Anything from work to preferred gym days, meal planning, and even mental health days.Use the "Key" box below to color code all your plans and activities. Think of it as a "YOU" calendar. Everything YOU need to do for yourself to be successful on this journey, plan it all out here.

S	M	T	W	T	F	S

KEY

MEAL PLANNING

This portion is for planning meals ahead. Come back here as often as you'd like
to plan your meals or even make grocery lists. You'll like to look back on this as well
throughout your journey to reflect on your mindset at the start of your journey.

	S	M	T	W
BREAKFAST				
LUNCH				
DINNER				
SNACKS				

MEAL PLANNING

T	F	S	SHOPPING LIST

WORKOUT LOG

	S	M	T	W	T	F	S
WEEK 1							
WEEK 2							
WEEK 3							
WEEK 4							

KEY

SLEEP TRACKER

31
30
29
28
27
26
25
24
23
22
21
20
19
18
17
16
15
14
13
12
11
10
9
8
7
6
5
4
3
2
1

6 7 8 9 10 11 12 1 2 3 4 5 6 7 8 9 10 11 12

MEAL TRACKER

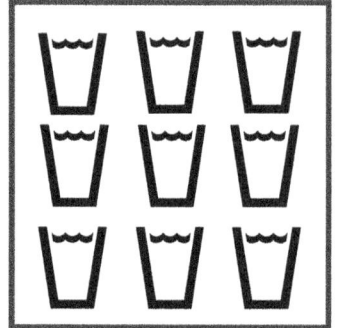

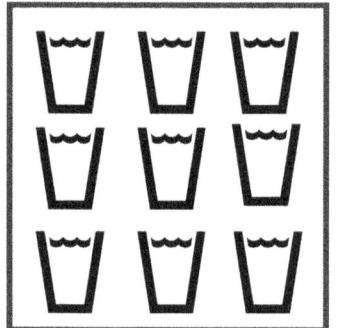

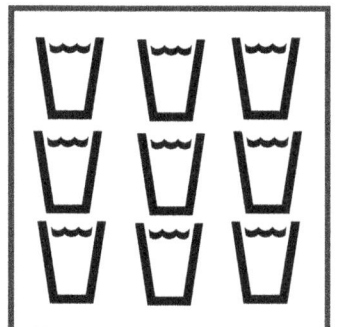

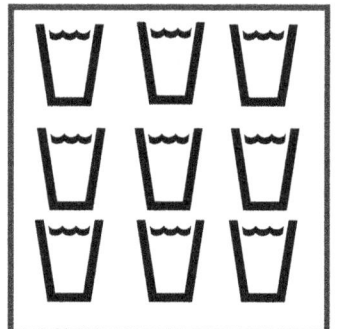

MEAL TRACKER

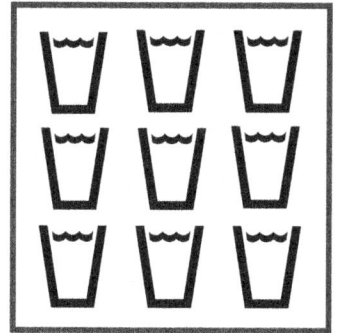

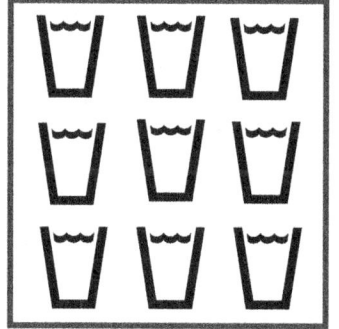

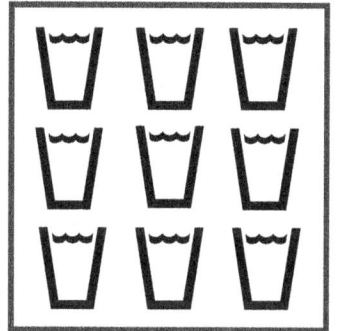

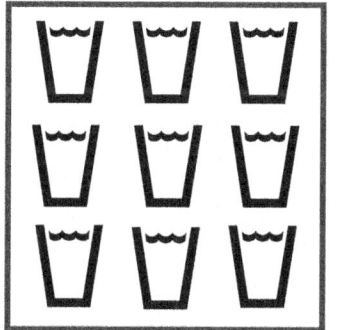

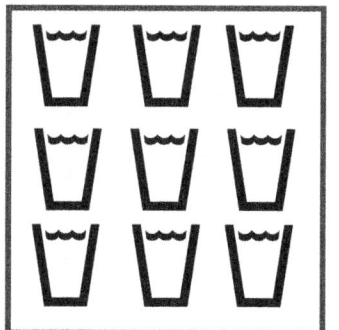

MEAL TRACKER

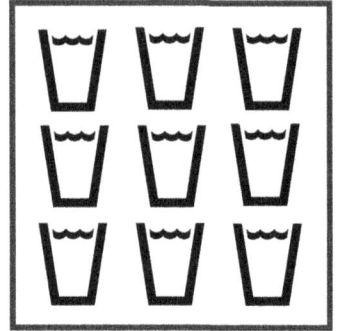

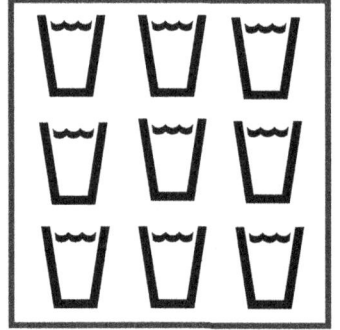

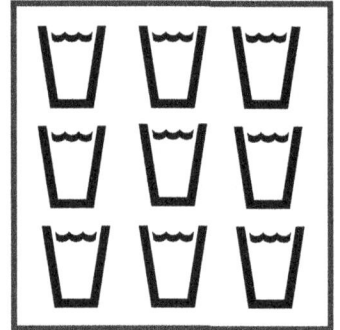

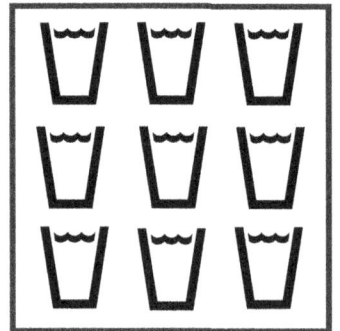

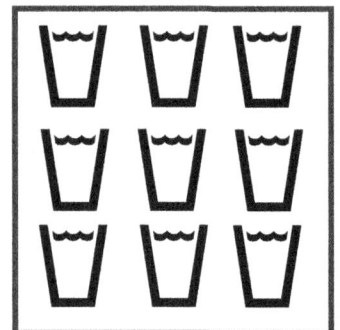

MEAL TRACKER

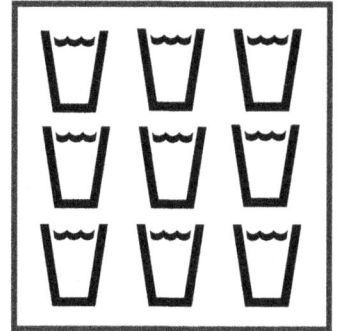

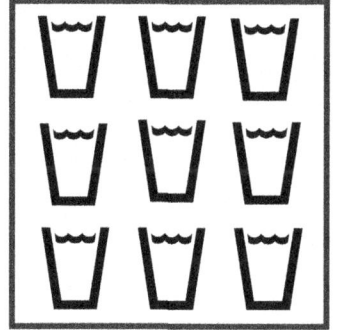

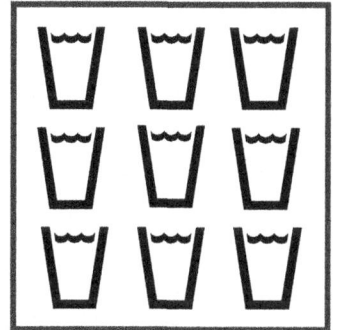

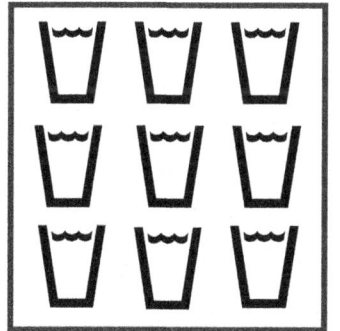

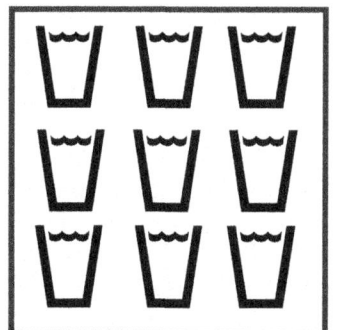

MEAL TRACKER

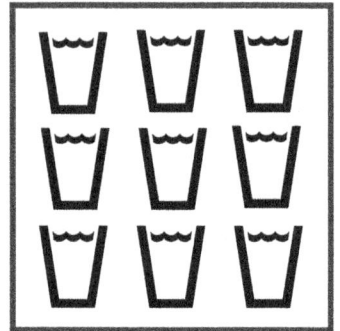

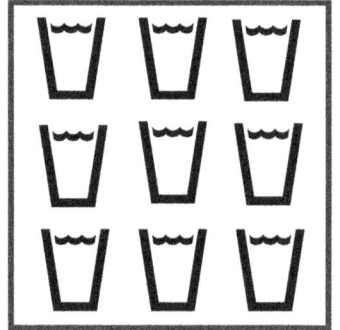

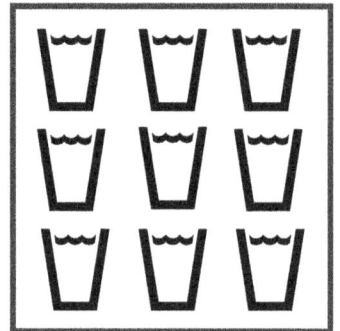

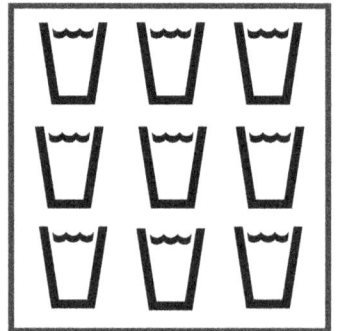

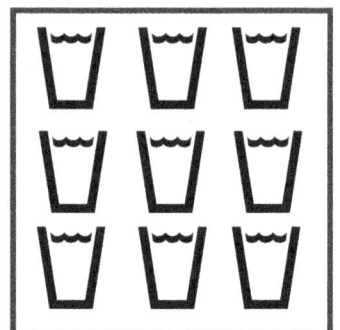

MEAL TRACKER

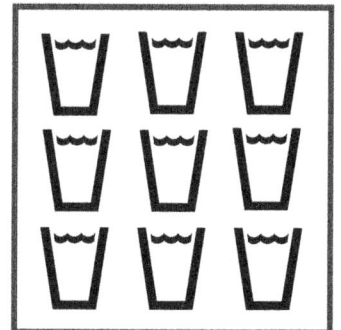

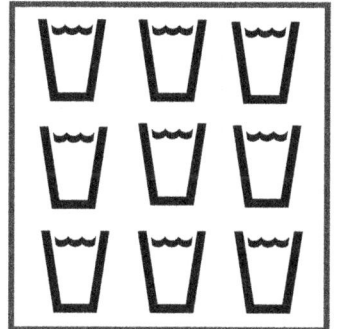

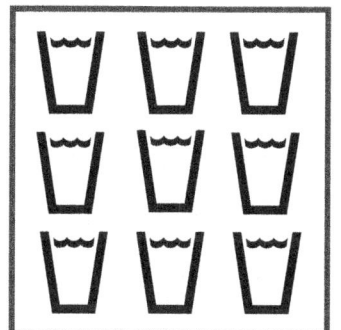

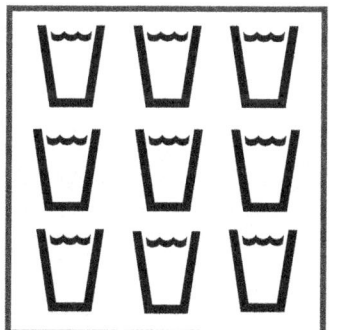

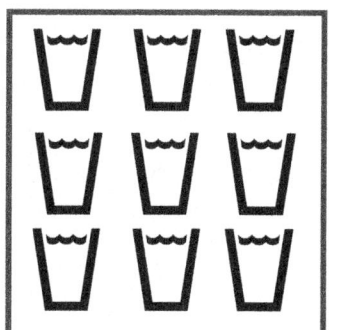

MEAL TRACKER

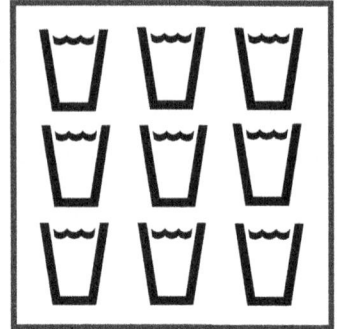

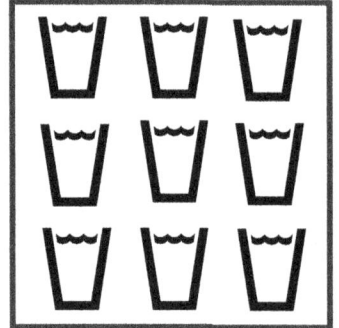

ROUND OVERVIEW

How many times did you eat fast food?

How many times did you cook your own meals?

Did you step out of your comfort zone with any meals?

How was your water intake?

What do you plan to change about your meals next round?

List 3 meals you'd like to cut out.

List 3 new meals you'd like to try.

ROUND OVERVIEW

DID YOU ACCOMPLISH YOUR GOAL WEIGHT? IF YES, WHAT DID YOU REWARD YOURSELF WITH AND WHY?

WERE YOU SUCCESSFUL IN CONTROLLING OR ENDING ANY BAD HABITS? WHICH HABITS DO YOU THINK WILL REQUIRE MORE OF YOUR TIME? DID YOU TAKE ON ANY GOOD HABITS? WHAT WERE THEY? WHAT HABITS ARE YOU INTERESTED IN WORKING ON NEXT ROUND?

HOW WERE YOUR MOODS THIS MONTH? WHAT HAVE YOU DONE FOR YOURSELF? HOW DO YOU FEEL AFTER COMPLETING THIS ROUND?

HOW'D THE SELF CARE REMINDER GO? HOW MANY TIMES DID YOU CATER TO YOURSELF? WHAT DO YOU HAVE PLANNED TO TREAT YOURSELF NEXT ROUND?

DID YOU TRY MEAL PLANNING THIS MONTH? DISCOVER ANY NEW RECIPES OR FOODS YOU ENJOYED? CHOOSE A DAY THAT WOULD BE GOOD FOR YOU TO MEAL PREP FOR THE WEEK.

HOW ACTIVE WERE YOU THIS ROUND? WHAT WAS YOUR MOST FREQUENT ACTIVITY? HOW DO YOU PLAN TO BE MORE ACTIVE NEXT ROUND? ANYTHING NEW YOU'D LIKE TO TRY?

WHAT DID YOUR SLEEP TRACKER REVEAL? HOW HAS IT CHANGED? TRY ANY OF OF THE TIPS/EXERCISES? WHICH ONES WERE HELPFUL?

ROUND 4

DON'T STOP UNTIL YOU'RE PROUD.

You never fail until
you stop trying.

Albert Einstein

FRIENDS + FAMILY

☐
☐
☐

CAREER

☐
☐
☐

LOVE

☐
☐
☐

FUTURE

☐
☐
☐

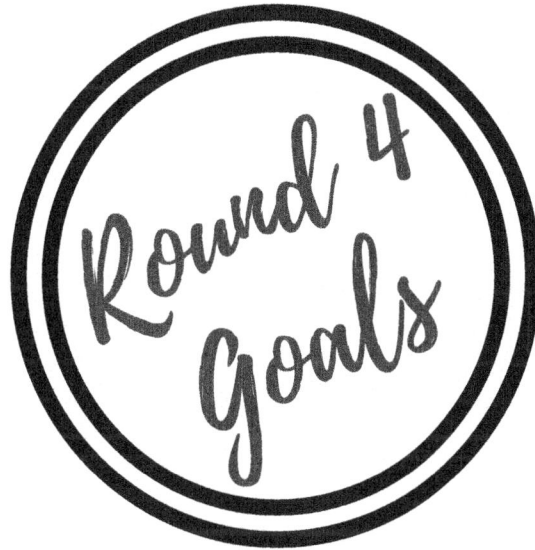

Round 4 Goals

FUTURE

☐
☐
☐

EXPERIENCES

☐
☐
☐

SELF CARE

☐
☐
☐

GETTING TO KNOW YOU

This portion is for you to get to know yourself a little better before we start the first round of your journey. You will do these every 3 rounds. It's a reflection that you'll be happy to look back on at the end of your yearlong journey. Write a short letter to yourself explaining who you are at this point in your life and what has inspired you to embark on this journey. Be honest with yourself. No one will read this but you. Don't overthink it. Just write freely.

HABIT TRACKER

Here is where you'll track your habits. In this round the dates are provided so jot down the name of the habit you are working towards or determined to break on the line below. (Ex: Fast food, Exercise, Smoking, etc.) Each day you are successful in either achieving or breaking this habit, you'll highlight or circle the date. The ultimate goal as you continue on through your rounds is to have the whole month colored in. The key is to break bad habits and enforce good ones.

1 2 3 4 5 6 7 8 9
10 11 12 13 14 15 16
17 18 19 20 21 22 23
24 25 26 27 28 29
30 31

_____

1 2 3 4 5 6 7 8 9
10 11 12 13 14 15 16
17 18 19 20 21 22 23
24 25 26 27 28 29
30 31

_____

1 2 3 4 5 6 7 8 9
10 11 12 13 14 15 16
17 18 19 20 21 22 23
24 25 26 27 28 29
30 31

_____

1 2 3 4 5 6 7 8 9
10 11 12 13 14 15 16
17 18 19 20 21 22 23
24 25 26 27 28 29
30 31

_____

MOOD TRACKER

Here is where you'll track your moods daily. Each round you will do this to track how you're feeling throughout your journey. In the "Key" box below, choose your moods and colors to represent them. Each day color in the hearts according to your mood. You're allowed to have good days and bad days. It's perfectly normal throughout your journey. It's called a journey for a reason, you aren't to be in the same place the entire time. Your health, mental state and appearance are all subject to change. Allow yourself to be human and allow yourself the necessary room to grow.

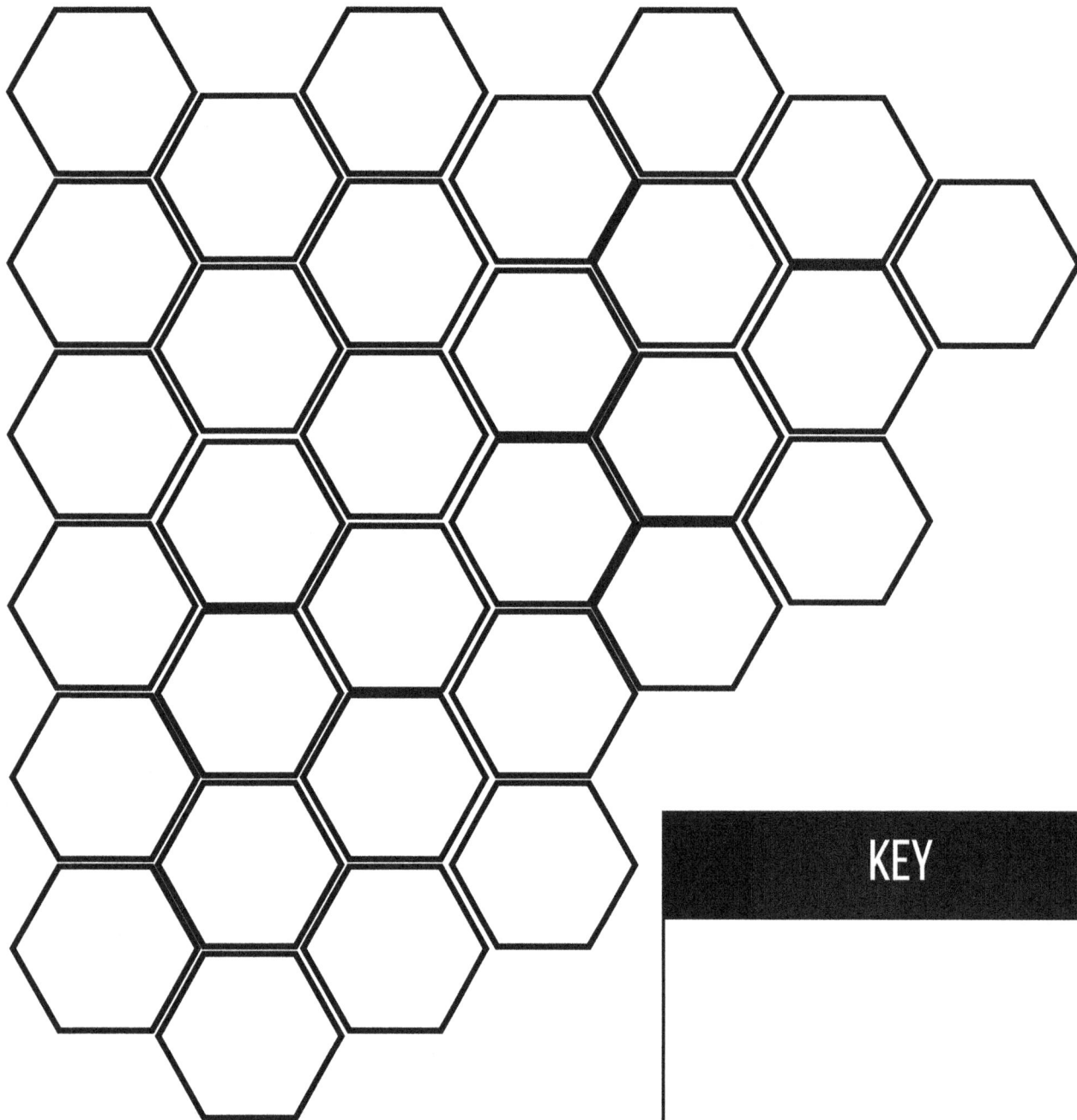

KEY

30 DAYS OF SELF CARE

For this portion you will list 30 acts of self care for each day this month. This is a challenge for you to spend a bit more time taking care of yourself. Be sure to include physical, mental and spiritual acts for the month. Cater to your overall health. When you've completed that task, come back and highlight it.

S	M	T	W	T	F	S

KEY

What Makes Me Happy?

This portion is a little different than the others. Here you will fill this page with ANY and EVERYTHING that makes you happy. This is a reflecting portion.

MENTAL HEALTH CHECK IN

This portion is a free write. Come back here as often as you'd like to pour out your feelings of how your journey is going. Some days are much harder than others and its helpful to get it out your head and jot it down. Just a few minutes a day, take a moment to free your mind here. You'll like to look back on this as well throughout your journey to reflect on your mindset at the start of your journey.

GRATITUDE LOG

This portion is a free write. Come back here as often as you'd like to pour out your feelings of gratitude during this round. You'll like to look back on this as well throughout your journey to reflect on your mindset at the start of your journey.

MONTH OVERVIEW

This undated calendar is for you to track and schedule activities.
Anything from work to preferred gym days, meal planning, and even mental health days. Use the
"Key" box below to color code all your plans and activities. Think of it as a "YOU" calendar.
Everything YOU need to do for yourself to be successful on this journey, plan it all out here.

S	M	T	W	T	F	S

KEY

MEAL PLANNING

This portion is for planning meals ahead. Come back here as often as you'd like to plan your meals or even make grocery lists. You'll like to look back on this as well throughout your journey to reflect on your mindset at the start of your journey.

	S	M	T	W
BREAKFAST				
LUNCH				
DINNER				
SNACKS				

MEAL PLANNING

T	F	S	SHOPPING LIST

MOTIVATIONAL QUOTES

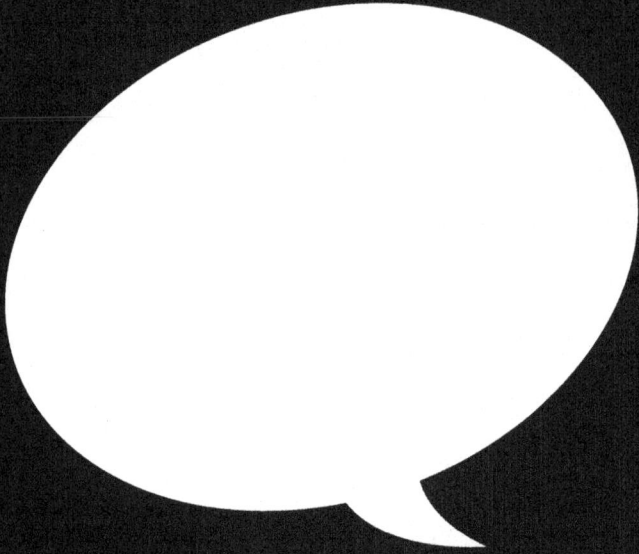

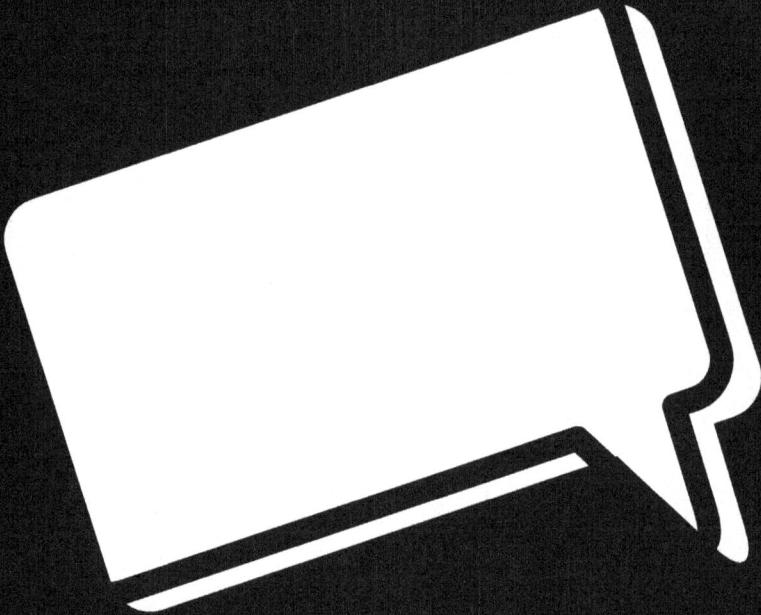
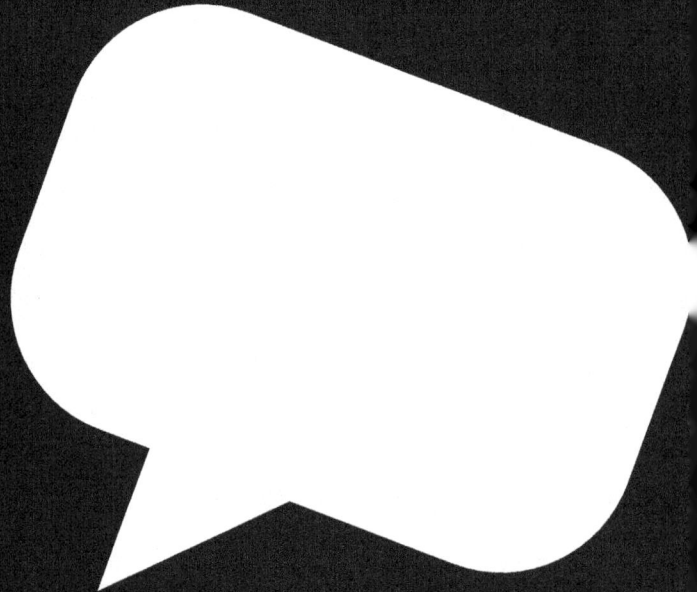
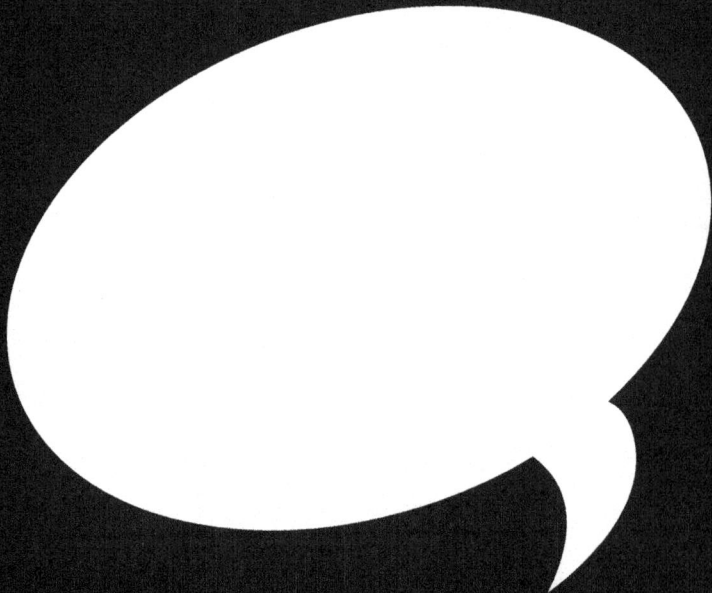
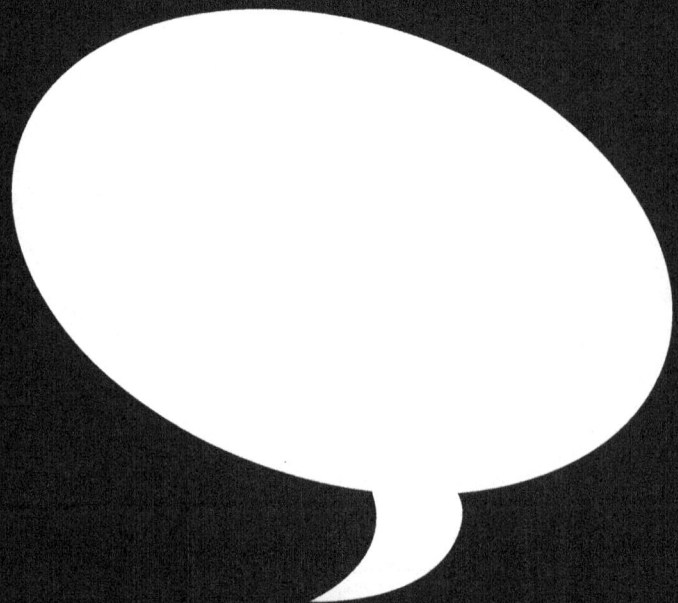

WORKOUT LOG

	S	M	T	W	T	F	S
WEEK 1							
WEEK 2							
WEEK 3							
WEEK 4							

KEY

SLEEP TRACKER

31
30
29
28
27
26
25
24
23
22
21
20
19
18
17
16
15
14
13
12
11
10
9
8
7
6
5
4
3
2
1

6 7 8 9 10 11 12 1 2 3 4 5 6 7 8 9 10 11 12

MEAL TRACKER

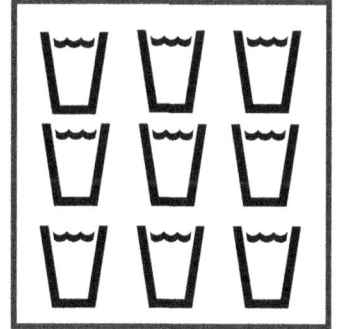

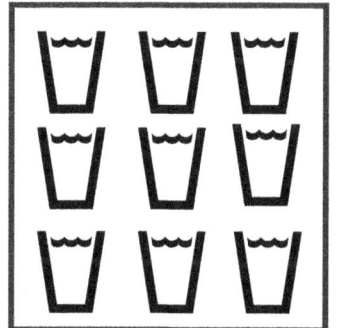

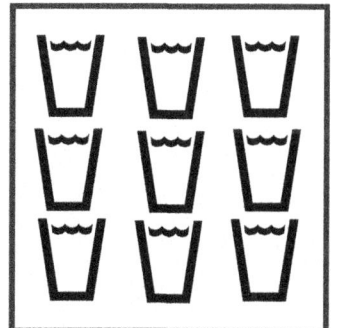

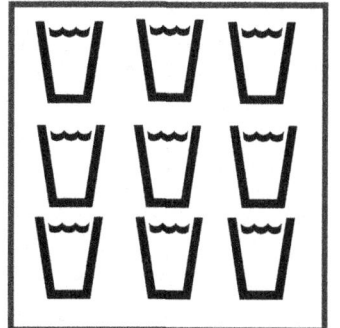

MEAL TRACKER

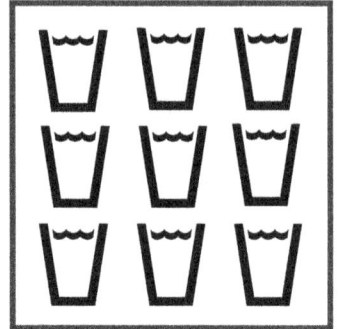

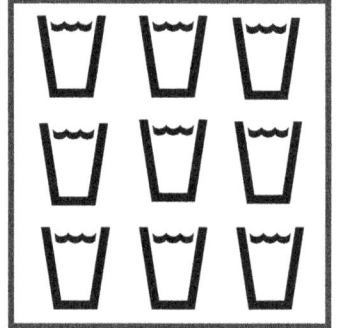

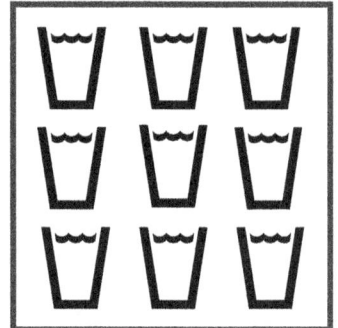

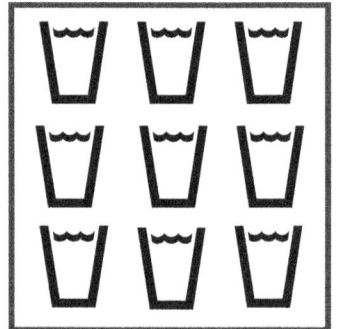

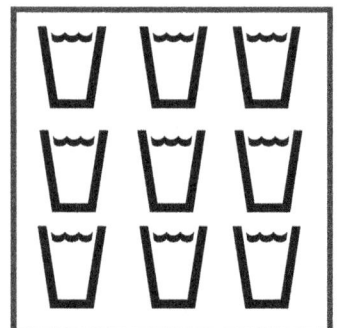

MEAL TRACKER

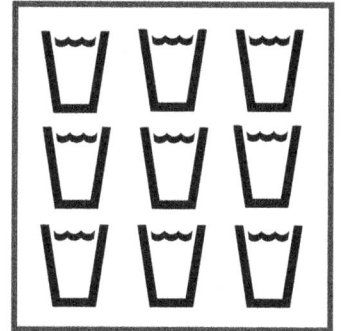

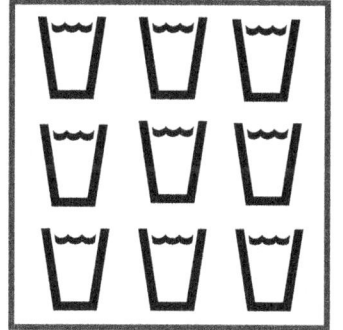

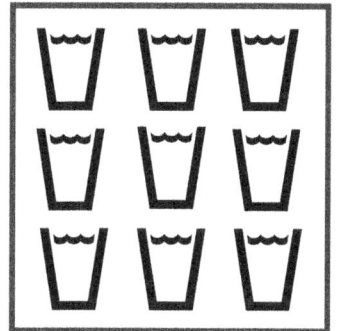

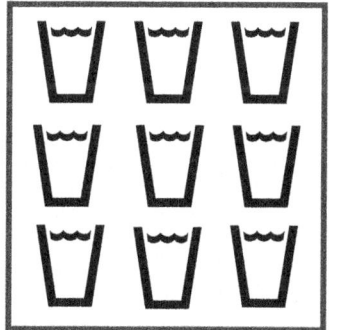

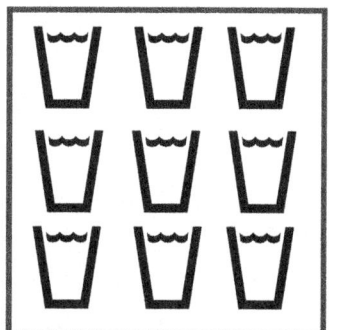

MEAL TRACKER

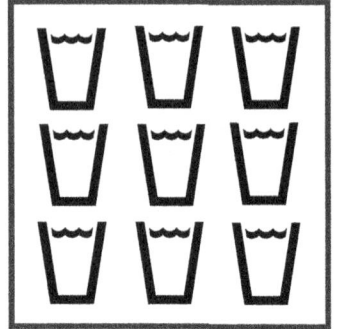

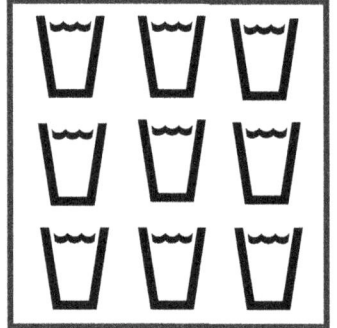

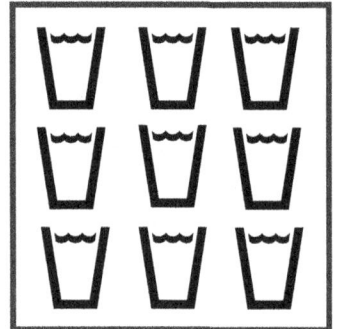

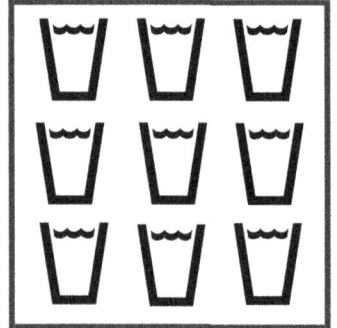

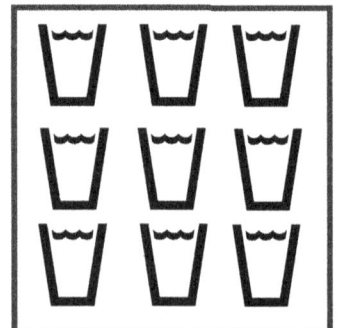

MEAL TRACKER

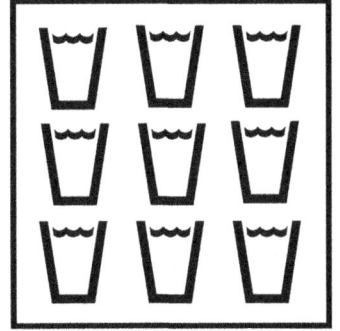

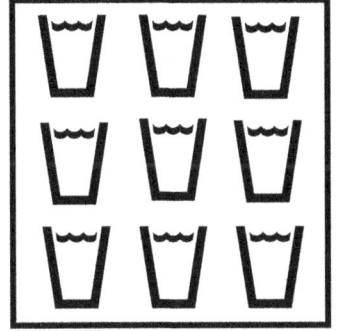

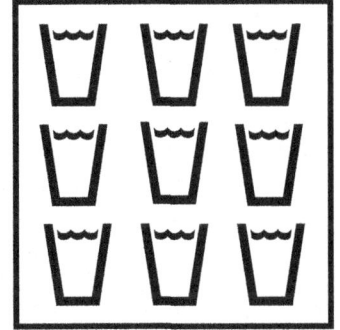

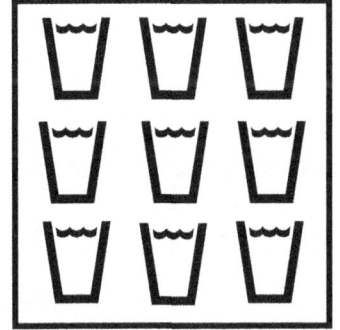

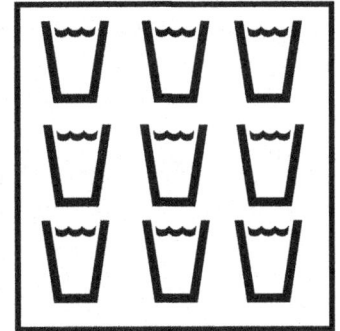

MEAL TRACKER

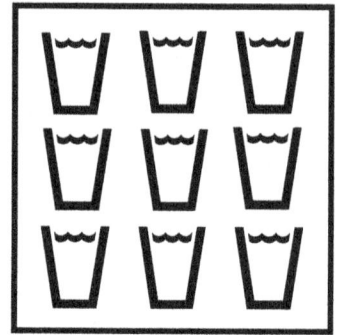

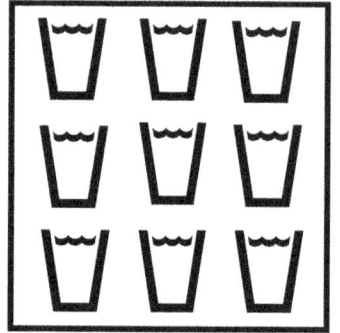

ROUND OVERVIEW

How many times did you eat fast food?

How many times did you cook your own meals?

Did you step out of your comfort zone with any meals?

How was your water intake?

What do you plan to change about your meals next round?

List 3 meals you'd like to cut out.

List 3 new meals you'd like to try.

ROUND OVERVIEW

DID YOU ACCOMPLISH YOUR GOAL WEIGHT? IF YES, WHAT DID YOU REWARD YOURSELF WITH AND WHY?

WERE YOU SUCCESSFUL IN CONTROLLING OR ENDING ANY BAD HABITS? WHICH HABITS DO YOU THINK WILL REQUIRE MORE OF YOUR TIME? DID YOU TAKE ON ANY GOOD HABITS? WHAT WERE THEY? WHAT HABITS ARE YOU INTERESTED IN WORKING ON NEXT ROUND?

HOW WERE YOUR MOODS THIS MONTH? WHAT HAVE YOU DONE FOR YOURSELF? HOW DO YOU FEEL AFTER COMPLETING THIS ROUND?

HOW'D THE SELF CARE REMINDER GO? HOW MANY TIMES DID YOU CATER TO YOURSELF? WHAT DO YOU HAVE PLANNED TO TREAT YOURSELF NEXT ROUND?

DID YOU TRY MEAL PLANNING THIS MONTH? DISCOVER ANY NEW RECIPES OR FOODS YOU ENJOYED? CHOOSE A DAY THAT WOULD BE GOOD FOR YOU TO MEAL PREP FOR THE WEEK.

HOW ACTIVE WERE YOU THIS ROUND? WHAT WAS YOUR MOST FREQUENT ACTIVITY? HOW DO YOU PLAN TO BE MORE ACTIVE NEXT ROUND? ANYTHING NEW YOU'D LIKE TO TRY?

WHAT DID YOUR SLEEP TRACKER REVEAL? HOW HAS IT CHANGED? TRY ANY OF OF THE TIPS/EXERCISES? WHICH ONES WERE HELPFUL?

ROUND 5

YOUR ONLY LIMIT IS YOUR YOU.

The comeback is
always stronger
than the setback.
Unknown

ROUND 5 GOALS

HABIT TRACKER

Here is where you'll track your habits. In this round the dates are provided so jot down the name of the habit you are working towards or determined to break on the line below. (Ex: Fast food, Exercise, Smoking, etc.) Each day you are successful in either achieving or breaking this habit, you'll highlight or circle the date. The ultimate goal as you continue on through your rounds is to have the whole month colored in. The key is to break bad habits and enforce good ones.

1 2 3 4 5 6 7 8 9
10 11 12 13 14 15 16
17 18 19 20 21 22 23
24 25 26 27 28 29
30 31

_____

1 2 3 4 5 6 7 8 9
10 11 12 13 14 15 16
17 18 19 20 21 22 23
24 25 26 27 28 29
30 31

_____

1 2 3 4 5 6 7 8 9
10 11 12 13 14 15 16
17 18 19 20 21 22 23
24 25 26 27 28 29
30 31

_____

1 2 3 4 5 6 7 8 9
10 11 12 13 14 15 16
17 18 19 20 21 22 23
24 25 26 27 28 29
30 31

_____

MOOD TRACKER

Here is where you'll track your moods daily. Each round you will do this to track how you're feeling throughout your journey. In the "Key" box below, choose your moods and colors to represent them. Each day color in the hearts according to your mood. You're allowed to have good days and bad days. It's perfectly normal throughout your journey. It's called a journey for a reason, you aren't to be in the same place the entire time. Your health, mental state and appearance are all subject to change. Allow yourself to be human and allow yourself the necessary room to grow.

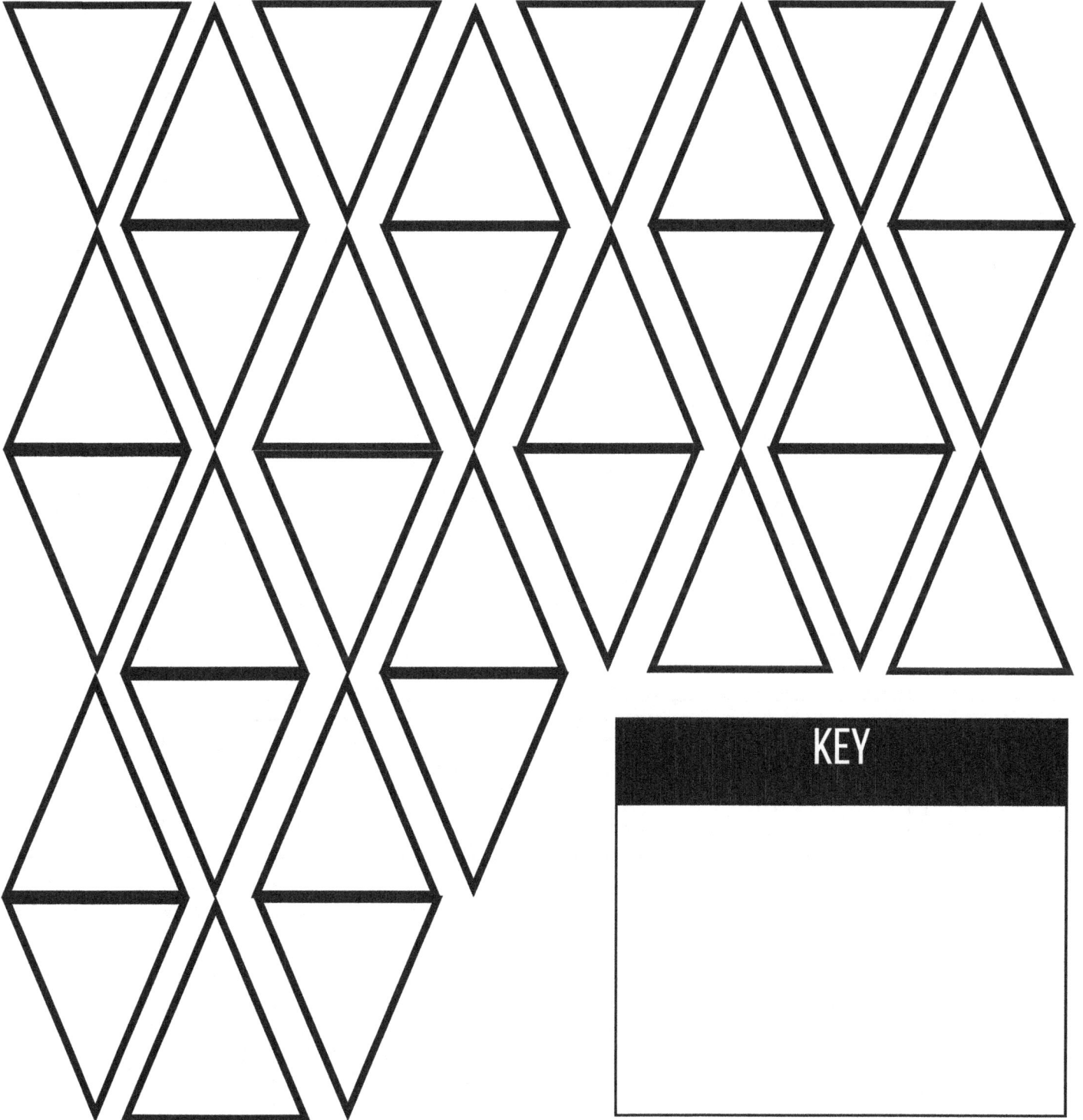

KEY

30 DAYS OF SELF CARE

For this portion you will list 30 acts of self care for each day this month. This is a challenge for you to spend a bit more time taking care of yourself. Be sure to include physical, mental and spiritual acts for the month. Cater to your overall health. When you've completed that task, come back and highlight it.

S	M	T	W	T	F	S

KEY

MENTAL HEALTH CHECK IN

This portion is a free write. Come back here as often as you'd like to pour out your feelings of how your journey is going. Some days are much harder than others and its helpful to get it out your head and jot it down. Just a few minutes a day, take a moment to free your mind here. You'll like to look back on this as well throughout your journey to reflect on your mindset at the start of your journey.

GRATITUDE LOG

This portion is a free write. Come back here as often as you'd like to pour out your feelings of gratitude during this round. You'll like to look back on this as well throughout your journey to reflect on your mindset at the start of your journey.

MONTH OVERVIEW

This undated calendar is for you to track and schedule activities.
Anything from work to preferred gym days, meal planning, and even mental health days. Use the "Key" box below to color code all your plans and activities. Think of it as a "YOU" calendar. Everything YOU need to do for yourself to be successful on this journey, plan it all out here.

S	M	T	W	T	F	S

KEY

MEAL PLANNING

This portion is for planning meals ahead. Come back here as often as you'd like to plan your meals or even make grocery lists. You'll like to look back on this as well throughout your journey to reflect on your mindset at the start of your journey.

	S	M	T	W
BREAKFAST				
LUNCH				
DINNER				
SNACKS				

MEAL PLANNING

T	F	S	SHOPPING LIST

SLEEP TRACKER

31
30
29
28
27
26
25
24
23
22
21
20
19
18
17
16
15
14
13
12
11
10
9
8
7
6
5
4
3
2
1

6 7 8 9 10 11 12 1 2 3 4 5 6 7 8 9 10 11 12

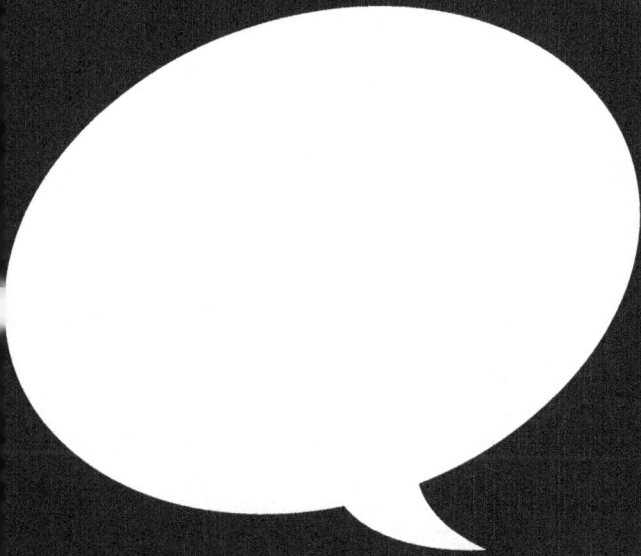

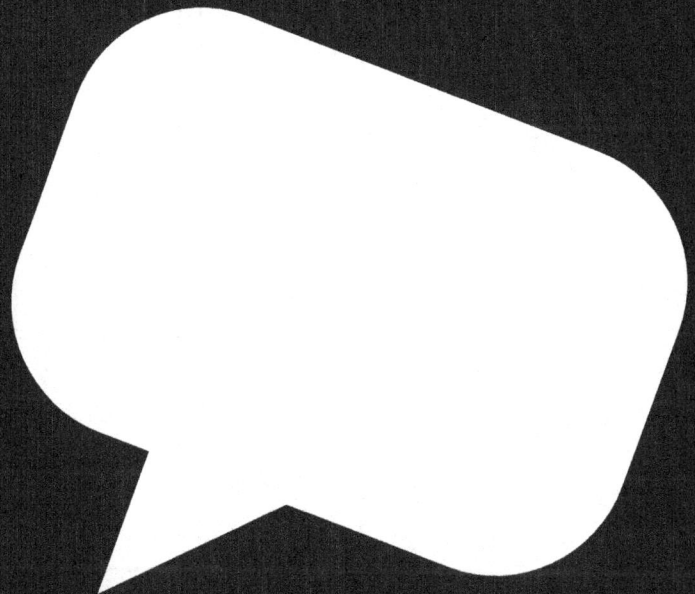
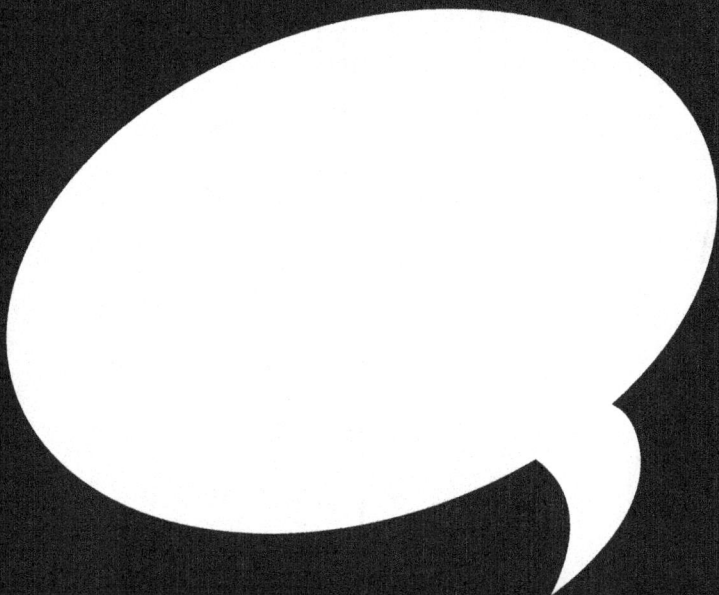
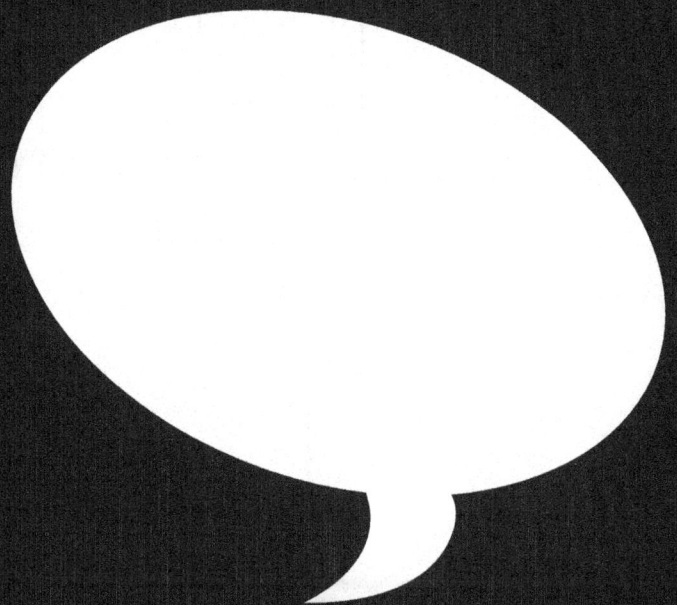

WORKOUT LOG

	S	M	T	W	T	F	S
WEEK 1							
WEEK 2							
WEEK 3							
WEEK 4							

KEY

MEAL TRACKER

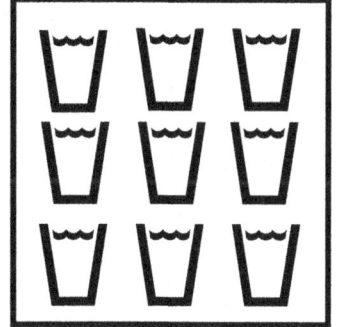

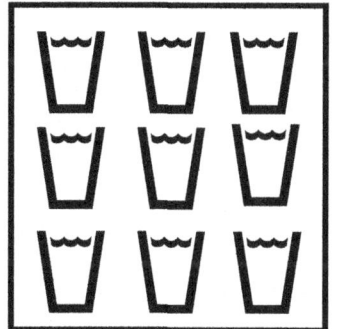

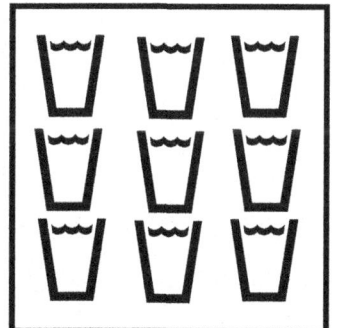

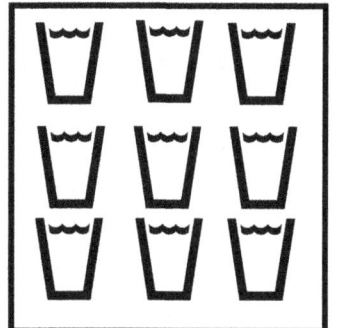

MEAL TRACKER

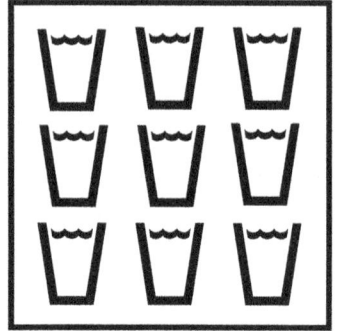

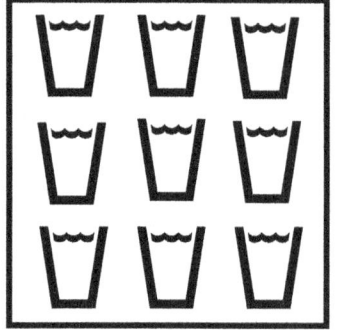

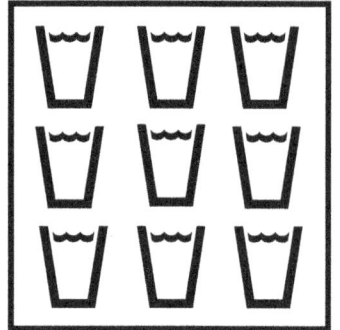

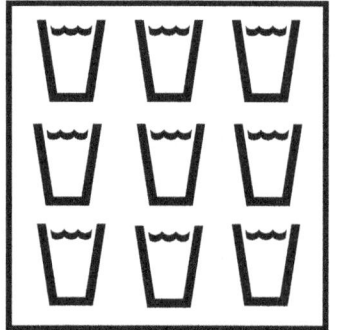

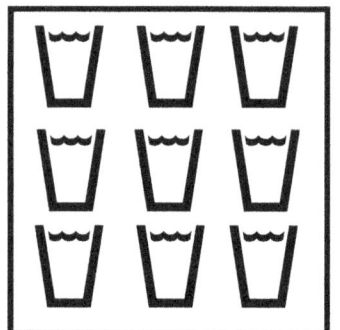

MEAL TRACKER

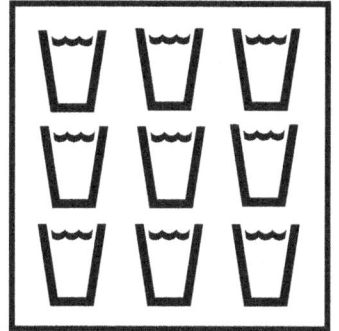

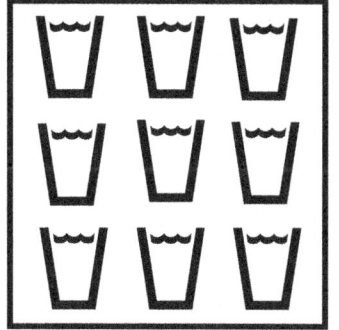

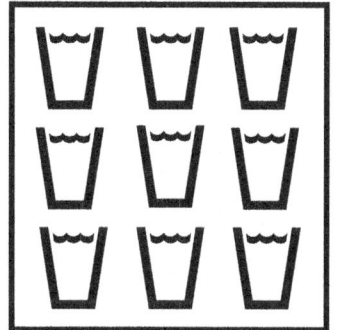

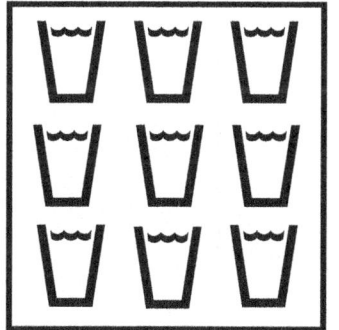

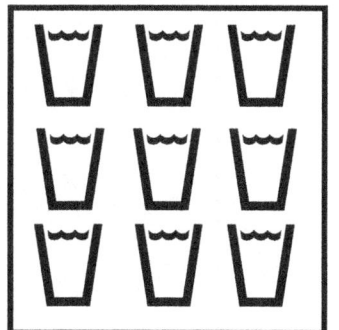

MEAL TRACKER

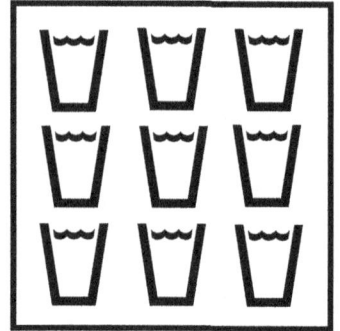

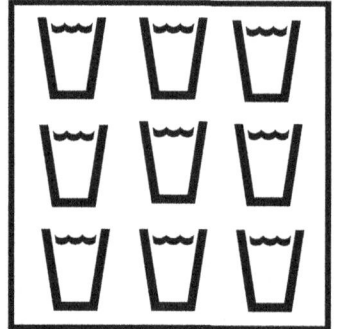

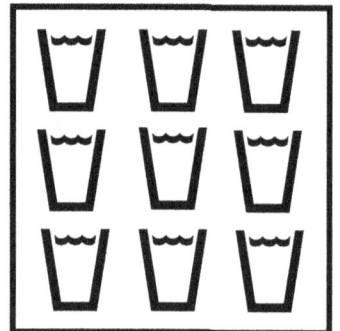

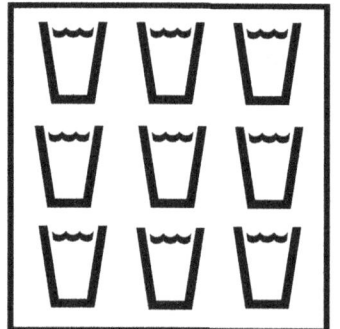

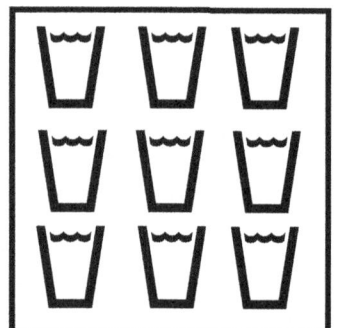

MEAL TRACKER

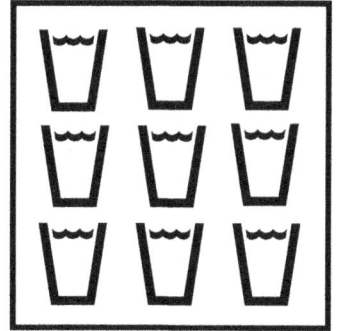

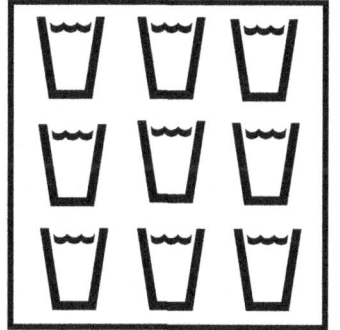

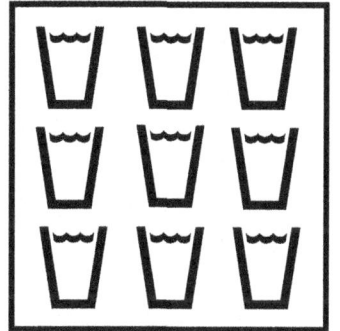

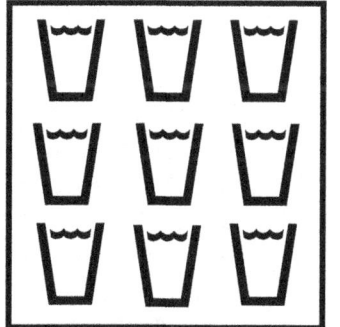

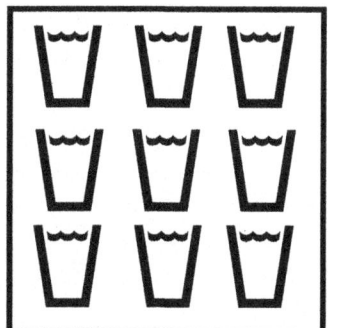

MEAL TRACKER

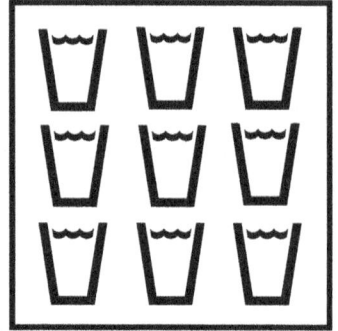

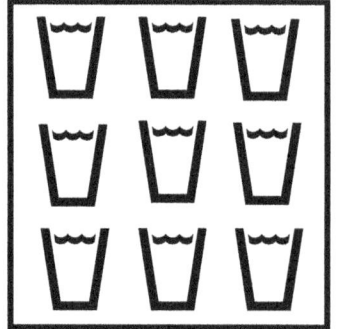

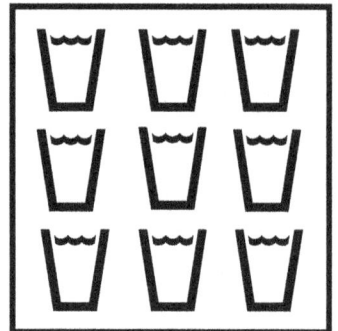

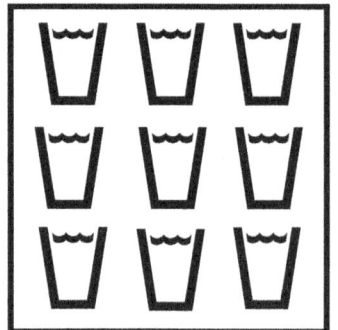

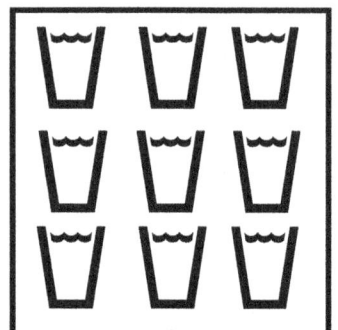

MEAL TRACKER

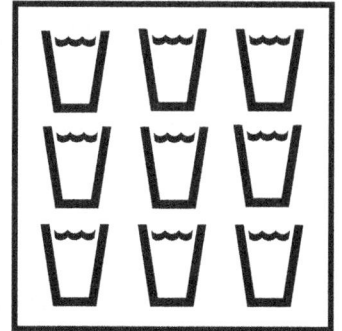

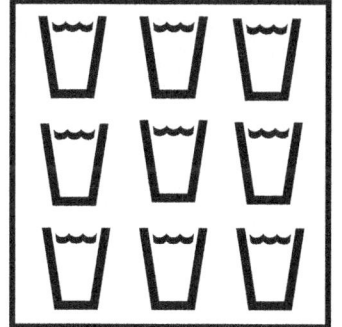

ROUND OVERVIEW

How many times did you eat fast food?

How many times did you cook your own meals?

Did you step out of your comfort zone with any meals?

How was your water intake?

What do you plan to change about your meals next round?

List 3 meals you'd like to cut out.

List 3 new meals you'd like to try.

ROUND OVERVIEW

DID YOU ACCOMPLISH YOUR GOAL WEIGHT? IF YES, WHAT DID YOU REWARD YOURSELF WITH AND WHY?

WERE YOU SUCCESSFUL IN CONTROLLING OR ENDING ANY BAD HABITS? WHICH HABITS DO YOU THINK WILL REQUIRE MORE OF YOUR TIME? DID YOU TAKE ON ANY GOOD HABITS? WHAT WERE THEY? WHAT HABITS ARE YOU INTERESTED IN WORKING ON NEXT ROUND?

HOW WERE YOUR MOODS THIS MONTH? WHAT HAVE YOU DONE FOR YOURSELF? HOW DO YOU FEEL AFTER COMPLETING THIS ROUND?

HOW'D THE SELF CARE REMINDER GO? HOW MANY TIMES DID YOU CATER TO YOURSELF? WHAT DO YOU HAVE PLANNED TO TREAT YOURSELF NEXT ROUND?

DID YOU TRY MEAL PLANNING THIS MONTH? DISCOVER ANY NEW RECIPES OR FOODS YOU ENJOYED? CHOOSE A DAY THAT WOULD BE GOOD FOR YOU TO MEAL PREP FOR THE WEEK.

HOW ACTIVE WERE YOU THIS ROUND? WHAT WAS YOUR MOST FREQUENT ACTIVITY? HOW DO YOU PLAN TO BE MORE ACTIVE NEXT ROUND? ANYTHING NEW YOU'D LIKE TO TRY?

WHAT DID YOUR SLEEP TRACKER REVEAL? HOW HAS IT CHANGED? TRY ANY OF OF THE TIPS/EXERCISES? WHICH ONES WERE HELPFUL?

ROUND 6

Goals

HABIT TRACKER

Here is where you'll track your habits. In this round the dates are provided so jot down the name of the habit you are working towards or determined to break on the line below. (Ex: Fast food, Exercise, Smoking, etc.) Each day you are successful in either achieving or breaking this habit, you'll highlight or circle the date. The ultimate goal as you continue on through your rounds is to have the whole month colored in. The key is to break bad habits and enforce good ones.

1 2 3 4 5 6 7 8 9
10 11 12 13 14 15 16
17 18 19 20 21 22 23
24 25 26 27 28 29
30 31

_____

1 2 3 4 5 6 7 8 9
10 11 12 13 14 15 16
17 18 19 20 21 22 23
24 25 26 27 28 29
30 31

_____

1 2 3 4 5 6 7 8 9
10 11 12 13 14 15 16
17 18 19 20 21 22 23
24 25 26 27 28 29
30 31

_____

1 2 3 4 5 6 7 8 9
10 11 12 13 14 15 16
17 18 19 20 21 22 23
24 25 26 27 28 29
30 31

_____

MOOD TRACKER

Here is where you'll track your moods daily. Each round you will do this to track how you're feeling throughout your journey. In the "Key" box below, choose your moods and colors to represent them. Each day color in the hearts according to your mood. You're allowed to have good days and bad days. It's perfectly normal throughout your journey. It's called a journey for a reason, you aren't to be in the same place the entire time. Your health, mental state and appearance are all subject to change. Allow yourself to be human and allow yourself the necessary room to grow.

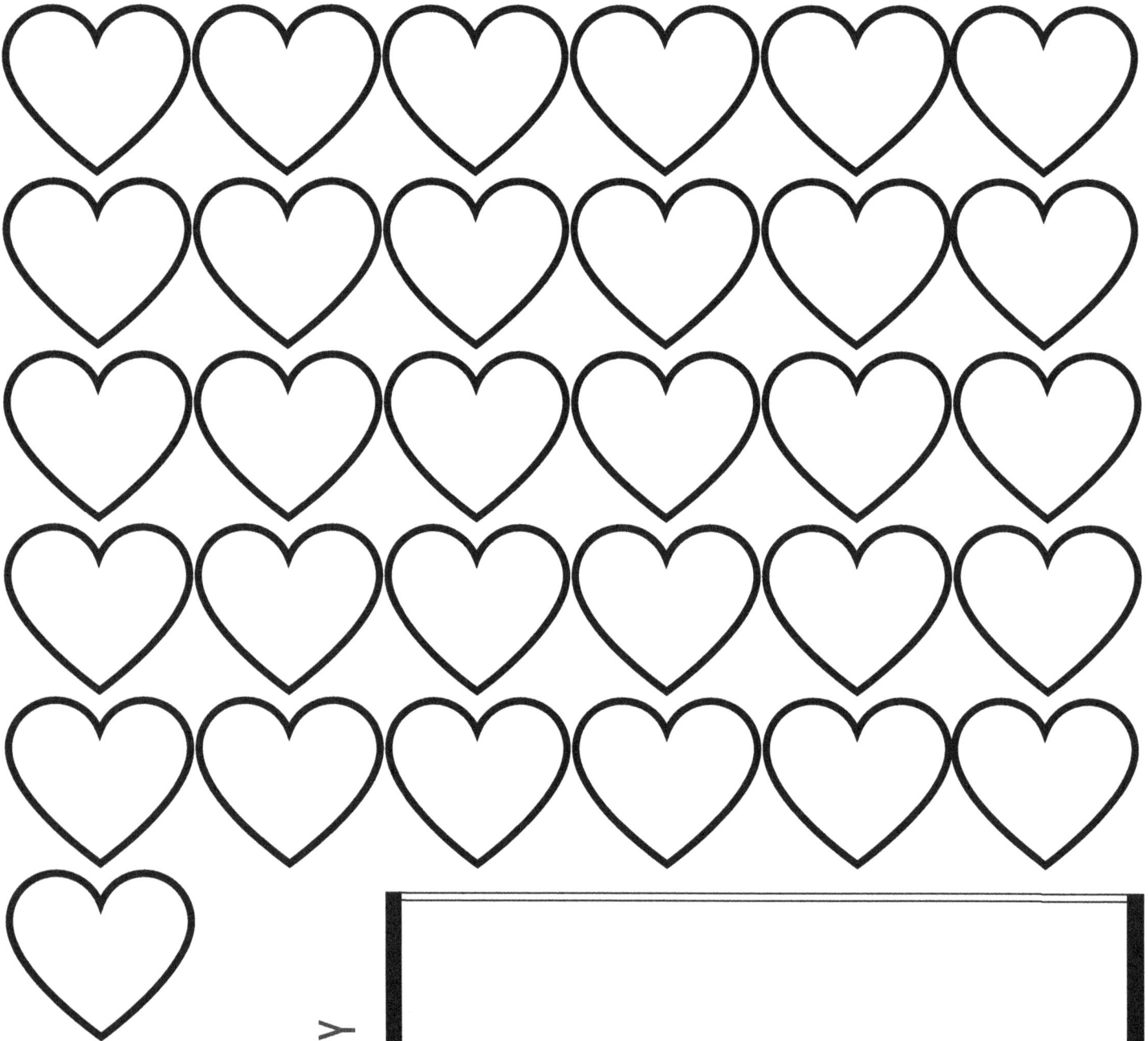

KEY

Self Care Reminder

This portion serves as a friendly reminder to take care of yourself. Fill this page up with things or activities you can do during this round that will cater to your mind, body and soul. Once these tasks have been completed, highlight them. Set aside time each week to do at least a few of these things, no matter how busy you are, pick a task, set a timer for 10-30 minutes and relax! You're halfway through your journey and you must recharge to keep pushing to the end!

MENTAL HEALTH CHECK IN

This portion is a free write. Come back here as often as you'd like to pour out your feelings of how your journey is going. Some days are much harder than others and its helpful to get it out your head and jot it down. Just a few minutes a day, take a moment to free your mind here. You'll like to look back on this as well throughout your journey to reflect on your mindset at the start of your journey.

GRATITUDE LOG

This portion is a free write. Come back here as often as you'd like to pour out your feelings of gratitude during this round. You'll like to look back on this as well throughout your journey to reflect on your mindset at the start of your journey.

MONTH OVERVIEW

This undated calendar is for you to track and schedule activities.
Anything from work to preferred gym days, meal planning, and even mental health days.
Use the "Key" box below to color code all your plans and activities. Think of it as a "YOU" calendar. Everything YOU need to do for yourself to be successful on this journey, plan it all out here.

S	M	T	W	T	F	S

KEY

MEAL PLANNING

This portion is for planning meals ahead. Come back here as often as you'd like to plan your meals or even make grocery lists. You'll like to look back on this as well throughout your journey to reflect on your mindset at the start of your journey.

	S	M	T	W
BREAKFAST				
LUNCH				
DINNER				
SNACKS				

MEAL PLANNING

T	F	S	SHOPPING LIST

PROGRESS TRACKER

This portion is a mid journey reflection how how many pounds you've lost/gained so far on this journey & how much closer you are to your goal! List the date your journey began, as well as your starting weight and goal weight! Then draw circles or hearts in the bottom jar, representing how many pounds you've already lost/gained and do the same in the top jar representing how many more pounds are left to reach your goal weight for this journey!

Start Date:

Starting Weight:

Goal Weight:

HOW MANY TO GO

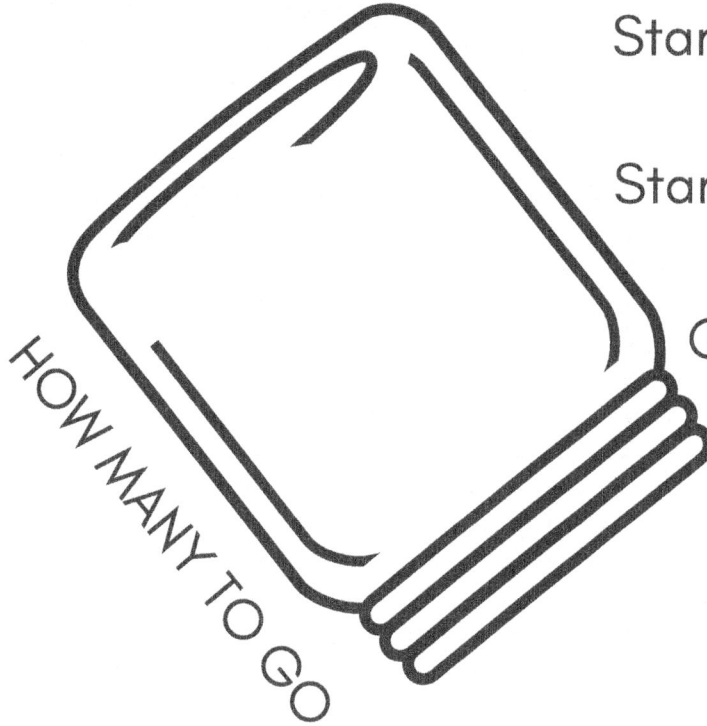

LITTLE by LITTLE, a LITTLE becomes a **LOT**

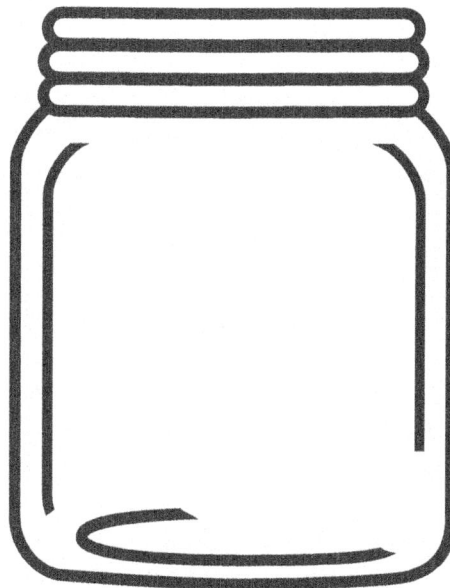

HOW MANY LOST/GAINED

SLEEP TRACKER

31
30
29
28
27
26
25
24
23
22
21
20
19
18
17
16
15
14
13
12
11
10
9
8
7
6
5
4
3
2
1

6 7 8 9 10 11 12 1 2 3 4 5 6 7 8 9 10 11 12

WORKOUT LOG

	S	M	T	W	T	F	S
WEEK 1							
WEEK 2							
WEEK 3							
WEEK 4							

KEY

MEAL TRACKER

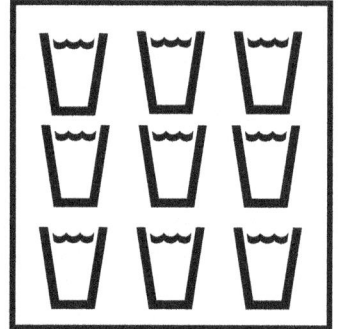

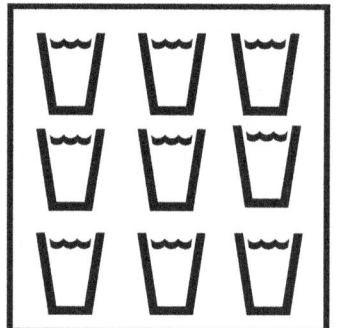

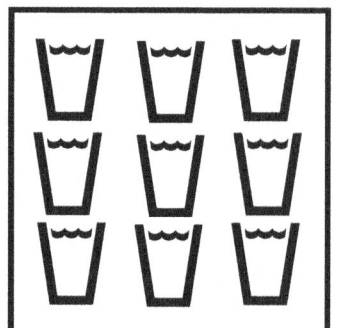

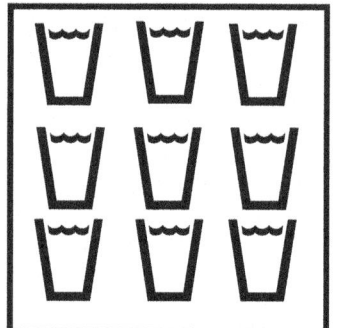

MEAL TRACKER

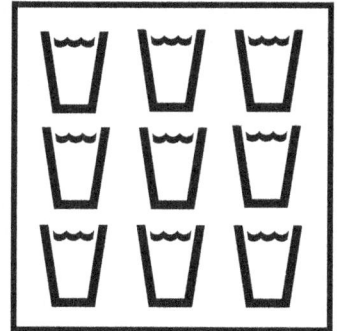

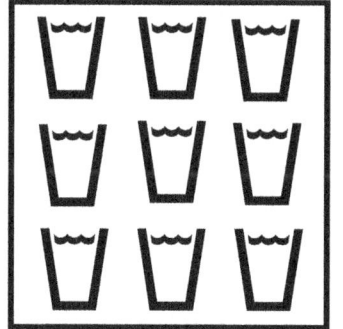

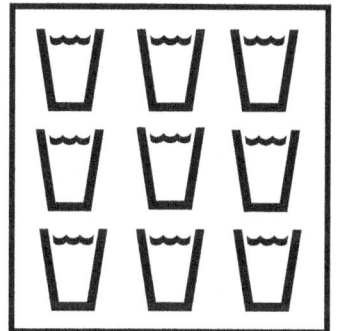

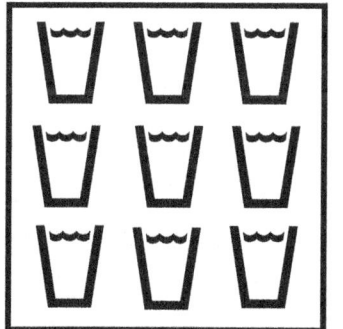

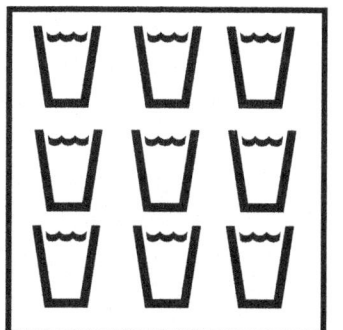

MEAL TRACKER

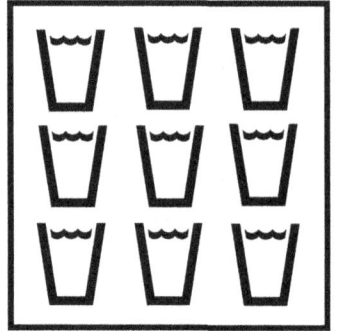

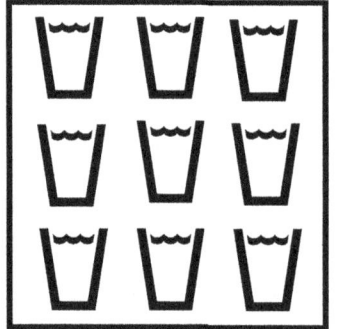

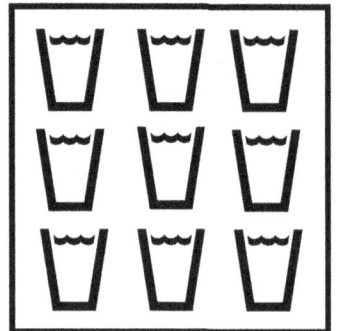

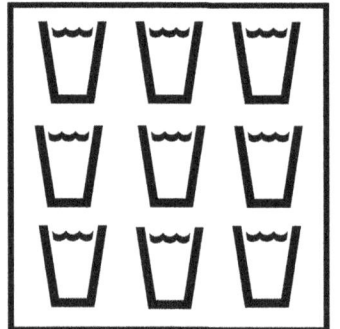

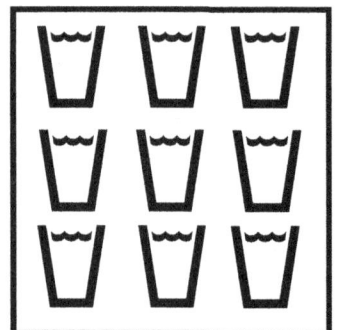

MEAL TRACKER

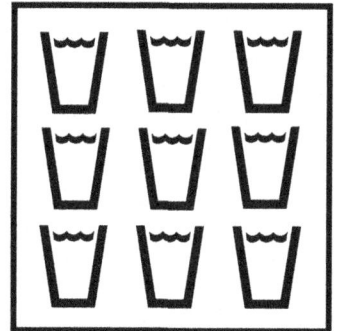

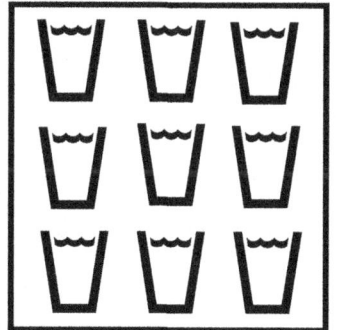

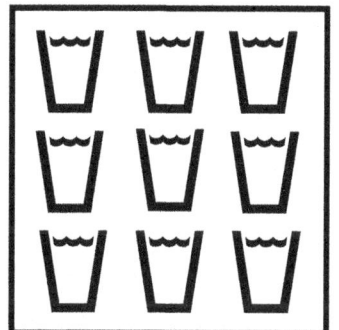

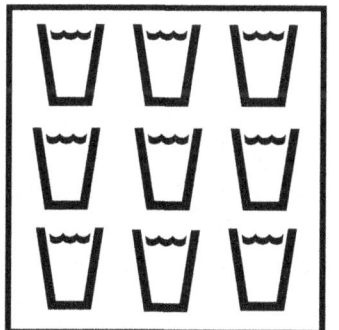

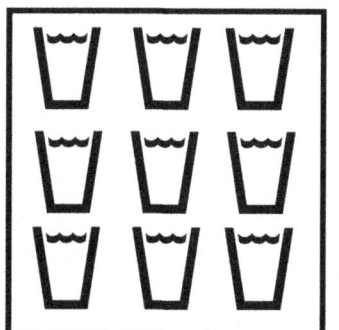

MEAL TRACKER

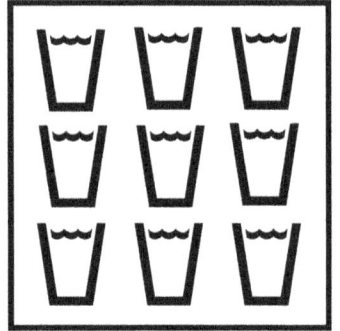

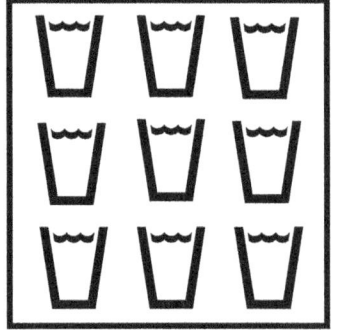

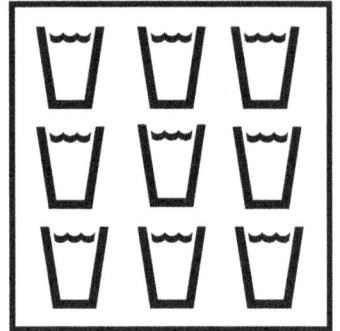

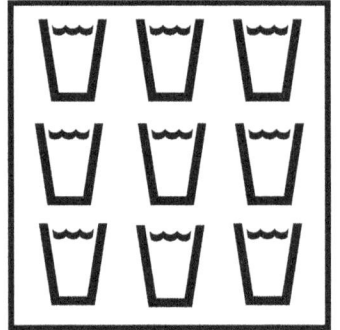

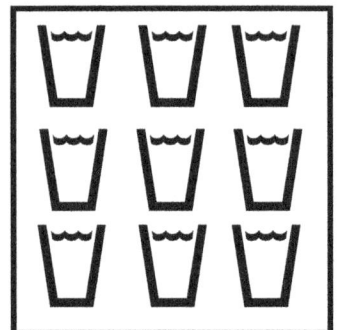

MEAL TRACKER

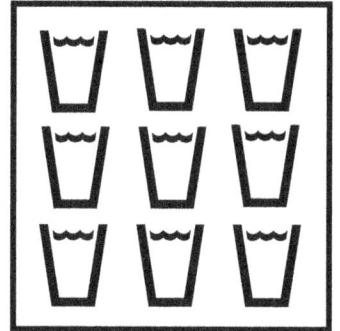

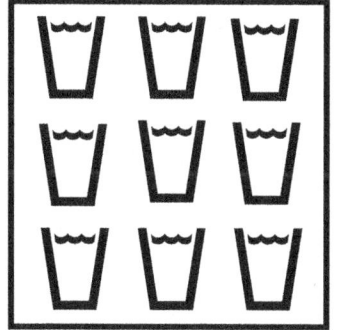

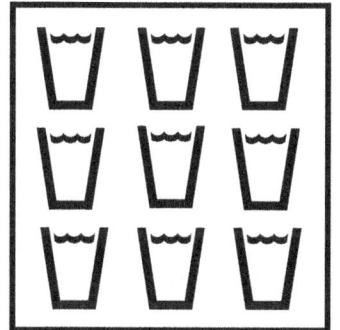

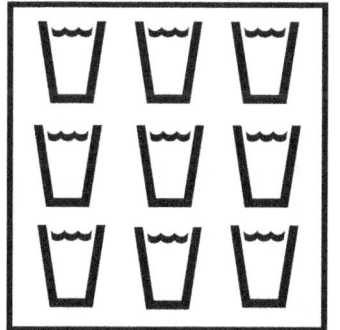

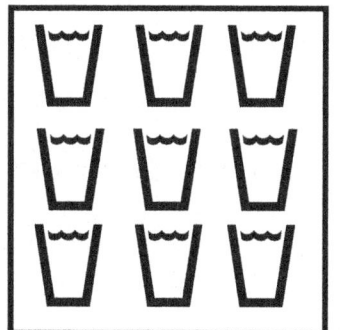

MEAL TRACKER

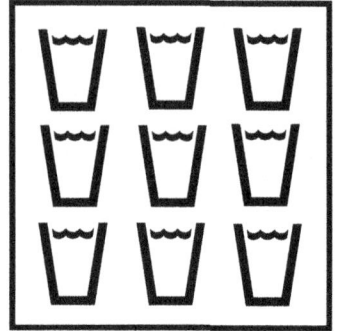

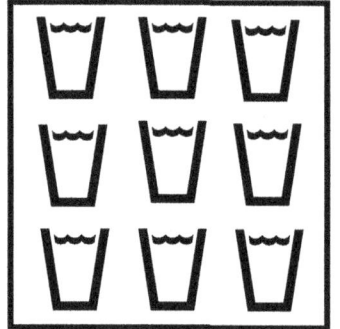

ROUND OVERVIEW

How many times did you eat fast food?

How many times did you cook your own meals?

Did you step out of your comfort zone with any meals?

How was your water intake?

What do you plan to change about your meals next round?

List 3 meals you'd like to cut out.

List 3 new meals you'd like to try.

ROUND OVERVIEW

DID YOU ACCOMPLISH YOUR GOAL WEIGHT? IF YES, WHAT DID YOU REWARD YOURSELF WITH AND WHY?

WERE YOU SUCCESSFUL IN CONTROLLING OR ENDING ANY BAD HABITS? WHICH HABITS DO YOU THINK WILL REQUIRE MORE OF YOUR TIME? DID YOU TAKE ON ANY GOOD HABITS? WHAT WERE THEY? WHAT HABITS ARE YOU INTERESTED IN WORKING ON NEXT ROUND?

HOW WERE YOUR MOODS THIS MONTH? WHAT HAVE YOU DONE FOR YOURSELF? HOW DO YOU FEEL AFTER COMPLETING THIS ROUND?

HOW'D THE SELF CARE REMINDER GO? HOW MANY TIMES DID YOU CATER TO YOURSELF? WHAT DO YOU HAVE PLANNED TO TREAT YOURSELF NEXT ROUND?

DID YOU TRY MEAL PLANNING THIS MONTH? DISCOVER ANY NEW RECIPES OR FOODS YOU ENJOYED? CHOOSE A DAY THAT WOULD BE GOOD FOR YOU TO MEAL PREP FOR THE WEEK.

HOW ACTIVE WERE YOU THIS ROUND? WHAT WAS YOUR MOST FREQUENT ACTIVITY? HOW DO YOU PLAN TO BE MORE ACTIVE NEXT ROUND? ANYTHING NEW YOU'D LIKE TO TRY?

WHAT DID YOUR SLEEP TRACKER REVEAL? HOW HAS IT CHANGED? TRY ANY OF OF THE TIPS/EXERCISES? WHICH ONES WERE HELPFUL?

MID JOURNEY REFLECTIONS

WHAT GOALS ARE YOU MOST PROUD OF ACCOMPLISHING SINCE STARTING YOUR JOURNEY?

REFLECTING ON BAD HABITS FROM ROUND 1, WHAT HABITS HAVE YOU ELIMINATED AND GAINED DURING THIS JOURNEY?

HOW HAVE YOUR MOODS BEEN OVER THE LAST 6 ROUNDS? DO YOU NOTICE IMPROVEMENTS? HAVE YOU BEEN DOING MORE ACTIVITIES & SPENDING TIME WITH THOSE WHO BRING YOU HAPPINESS?

HOW HELPFUL HAS THE MENTAL CHECK IN BEEN? DO YOU LOG FREQUENTLY?

HOW HELPFUL HAS THE GRATITUDE LOG BEEN? DO YOU LOG FREQUENTLY?

MID JOURNEY REFLECTIONS

CAN YOU SAY OVER THESE PAST 6 ROUNDS THAT YOU'VE MADE SELF CARE A PART OF YOUR ROUTINE? HOW OFTEN A WEEK ARE YOU SETTING TIME ASIDE TO PRACTICE SELF CARE?

HOW OFTEN HAVE YOU BEEN ACTIVE OVER THESE PAST 6 ROUNDS? HAVE YOU MADE BEING ACTIVE A PART OF YOUR ROUTINE? HOW DOES IT FEEL?

HOW HELPFUL HAS YOUR MANTRA BEEN? DO YOU RECITE IT DAILY? DO YOU HAVE IT MEMORIZED YET?

LIST A FEW WORDS OF ENCOURAGEMENT FOR YOURSELF DURING THE REMAINDER OF YOUR JOURNEY.

ROUND 7

DON'T LOOK BACK.

Old ways won't
open new doors.
Unknown

GOALS

HABIT TRACKER

Here is where you'll track your habits. In this round the dates are provided so jot down the name of the habit you are working towards or determined to break on the line below. (Ex: Fast food, Exercise, Smoking, etc.) Each day you are successful in either achieving or breaking this habit, you'll highlight or circle the date. The ultimate goal as you continue on through your rounds is to have the whole month colored in. The key is to break bad habits and enforce good ones.

1 2 3 4 5 6 7 8 9
10 11 12 13 14 15 16
17 18 19 20 21 22 23
24 25 26 27 28 29
30 31

_____

1 2 3 4 5 6 7 8 9
10 11 12 13 14 15 16
17 18 19 20 21 22 23
24 25 26 27 28 29
30 31

_____

1 2 3 4 5 6 7 8 9
10 11 12 13 14 15 16
17 18 19 20 21 22 23
24 25 26 27 28 29
30 31

_____

1 2 3 4 5 6 7 8 9
10 11 12 13 14 15 16
17 18 19 20 21 22 23
24 25 26 27 28 29
30 31

_____

MOOD TRACKER

Here is where you'll track your moods daily. Each round you will do this to track how you're feeling throughout your journey. In the "Key" box below, choose your moods and colors to represent them. Each day color in the hearts according to your mood. You're allowed to have good days and bad days. It's perfectly normal throughout your journey. It's called a journey for a reason, you aren't to be in the same place the entire time. Your health, mental state and appearance are all subject to change. Allow yourself to be human and allow yourself the necessary room to grow.

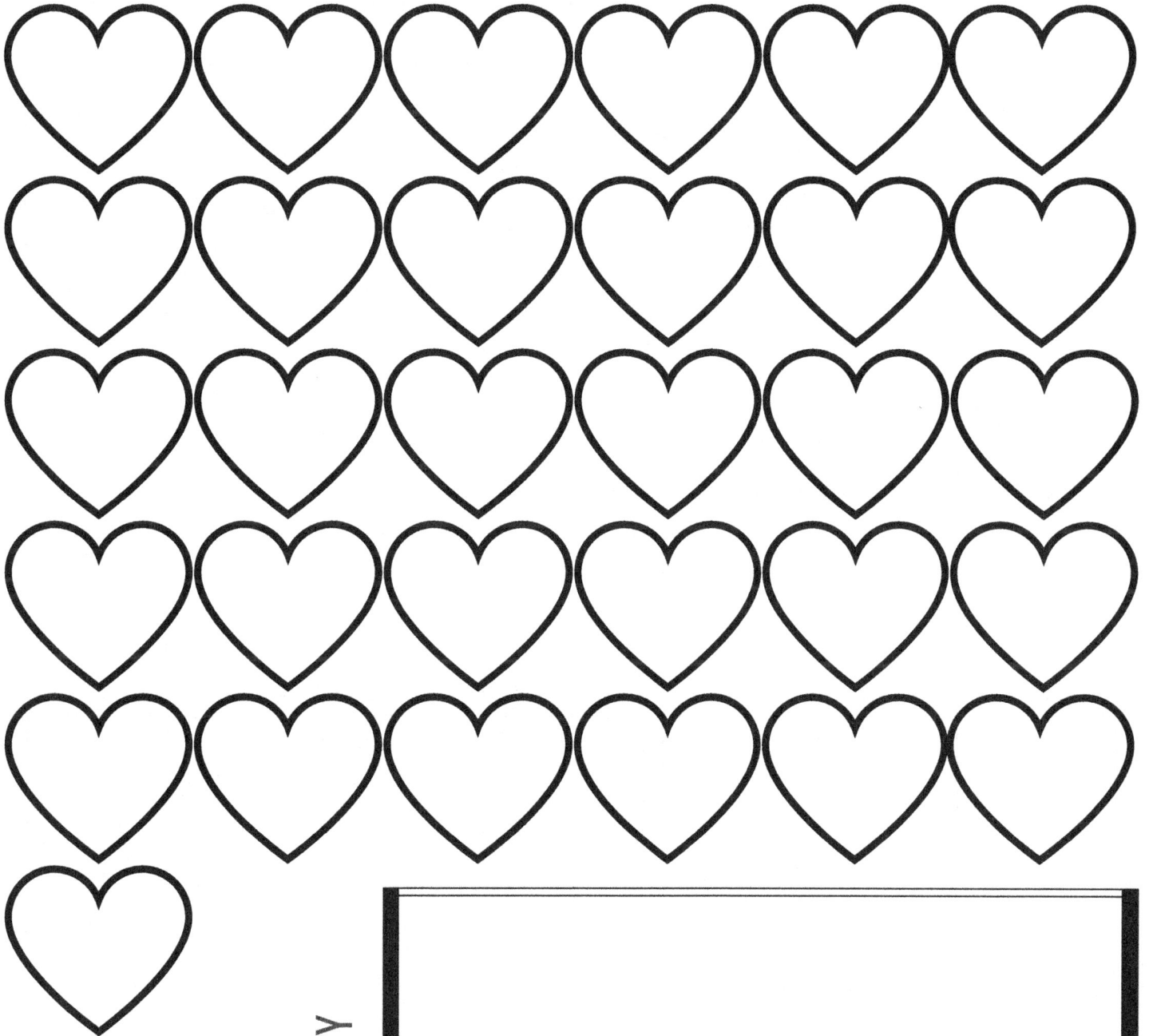

KEY

30 DAYS OF SELF CARE

For this portion you will list 30 acts of self care for each day this month. This is a challenge for you to spend a bit more time taking care of yourself. Be sure to include physical, mental and spiritual acts for the month. Cater to your overall health. When you've completed that task, come back and highlight it.

S	M	T	W	T	F	S

KEY

GETTING TO KNOW YOU

This portion is for you to get to know yourself a little better before we start the first round of your journey. You will do these every 3 rounds. It's a reflection that you'll be happy to look back on at the end of your yearlong journey. Write a short letter to yourself explaining who you are at this point in your life and what has inspired you to embark on this journey. Be honest with yourself. No one will read this but you. Don't overthink it. Just write freely.

MENTAL HEALTH CHECK IN

This portion is a free write. Come back here as often as you'd like to pour out your feelings of how your journey is going. Some days are much harder than others and its helpful to get it out your head and jot it down. Just a few minutes a day, take a moment to free your mind here. You'll like to look back on this as well throughout your journey to reflect on your mindset at the start of your journey.

GRATITUDE LOG

This portion is a free write. Come back here as often as you'd like to pour out your feelings of gratitude during this round. You'll like to look back on this as well throughout your journey to reflect on your mindset at the start of your journey.

MONTH OVERVIEW

This undated calendar is for you to track and schedule activities. Anything from work to preferred gym days, meal planning, and even mental health days. Use the "Key" box below to color code all your plans and activities. Think of it as a "YOU" calendar. Everything YOU need to do for yourself to be successful on this journey, plan it all out here.

S	M	T	W	T	F	S

KEY

MEAL PLANNING

This portion is for planning meals ahead. Come back here as often as you'd like to plan your meals or even make grocery lists. You'll like to look back on this as well throughout your journey to reflect on your mindset at the start of your journey.

	S	M	T	W
BREAKFAST				
LUNCH				
DINNER				
SNACKS				

MEAL PLANNING

T	F	S	SHOPPING LIST

SLEEP TRACKER

31
30
29
28
27
26
25
24
23
22
21
20
19
18
17
16
15
14
13
12
11
10
9
8
7
6
5
4
3
2
1

6 7 8 9 10 11 12 1 2 3 4 5 6 7 8 9 10 11 12

WORKOUT LOG

	S	M	T	W	T	F	S
WEEK 1							
WEEK 2							
WEEK 3							
WEEK 4							

KEY

MEAL TRACKER

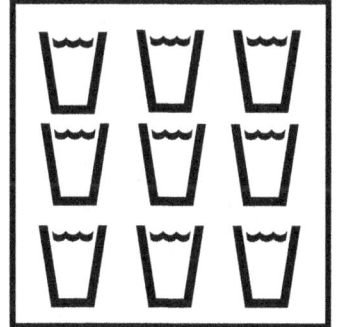

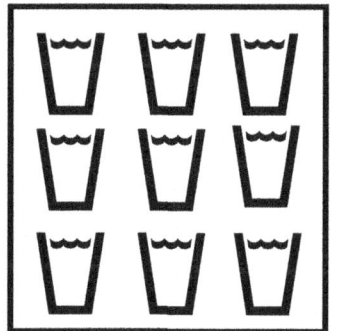

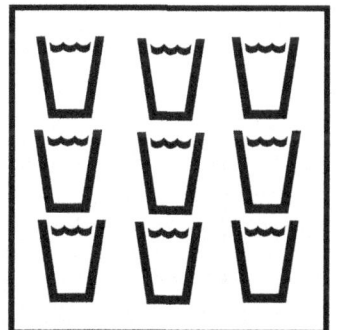

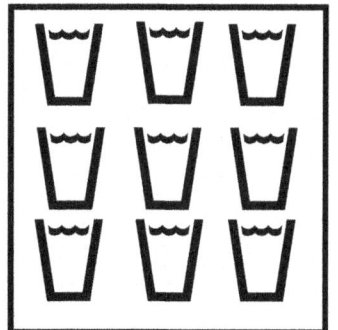

MEAL TRACKER

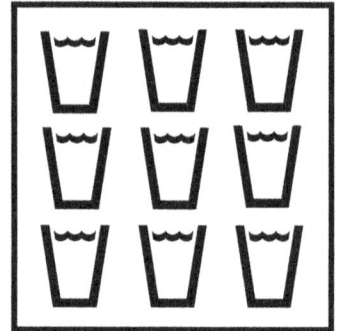

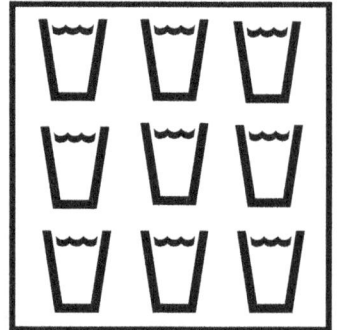

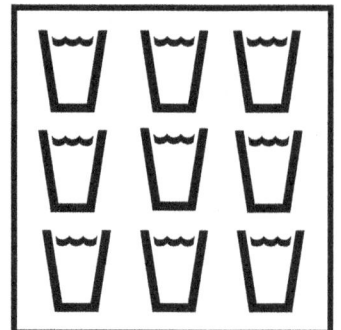

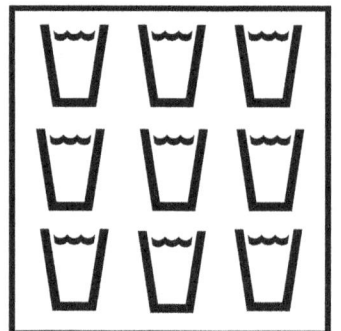

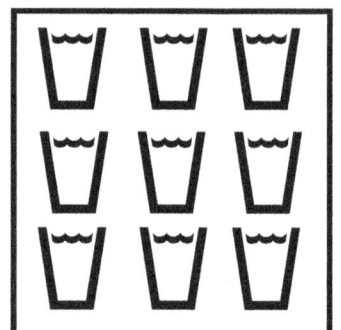

MEAL TRACKER

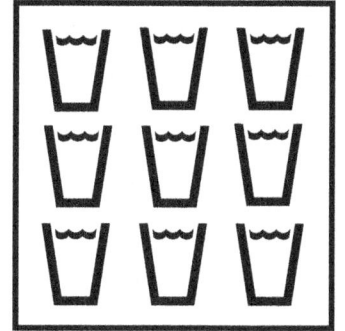

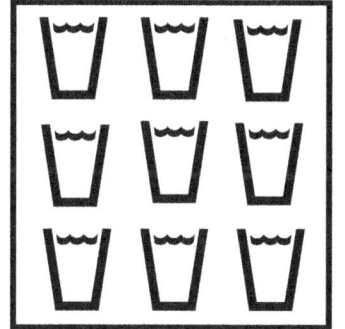

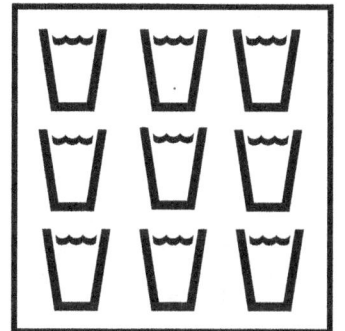

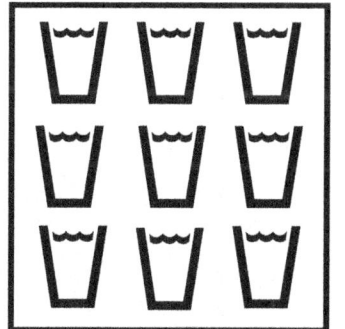

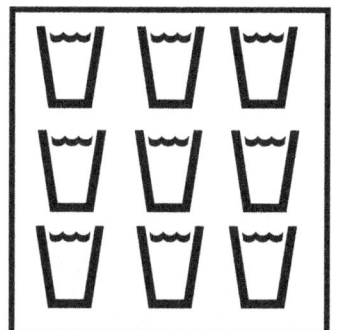

MEAL TRACKER

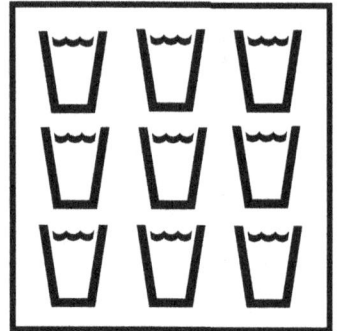

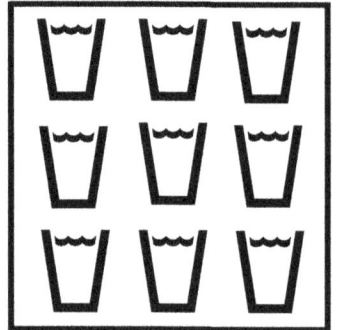

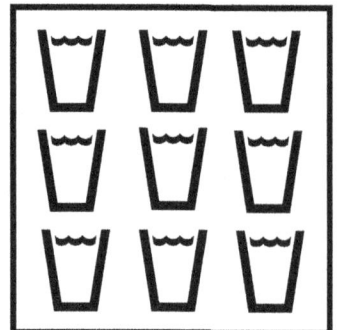

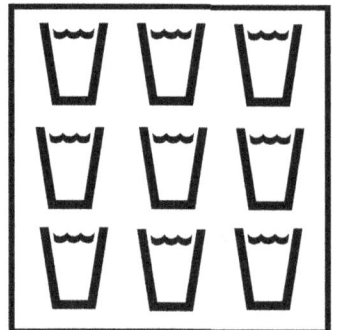

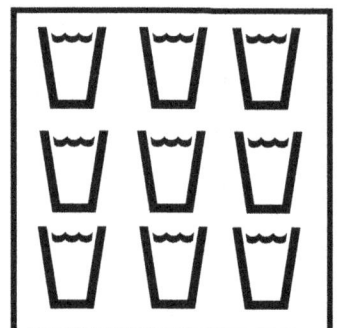

MEAL TRACKER

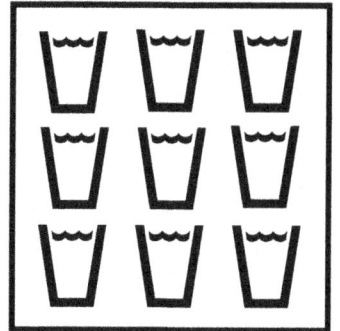

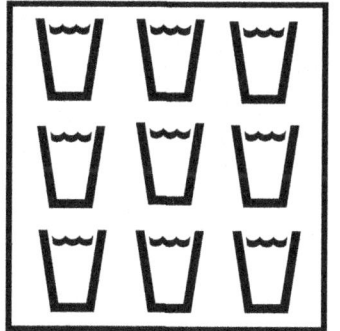

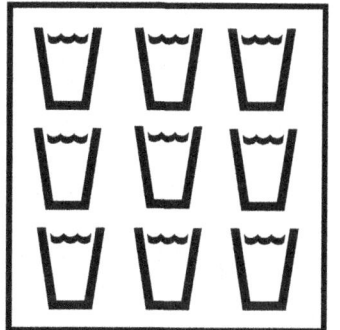

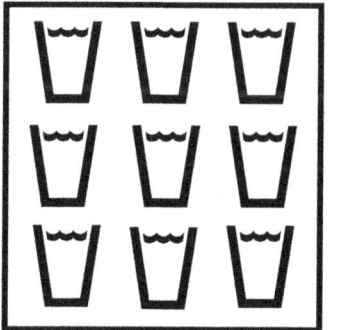

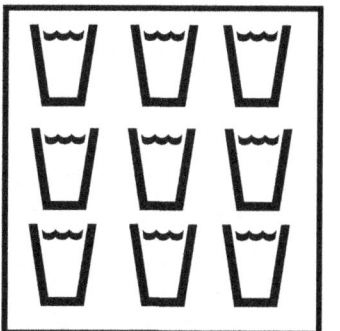

MEAL TRACKER

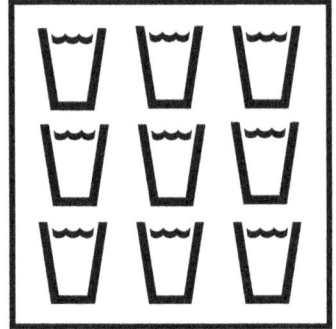

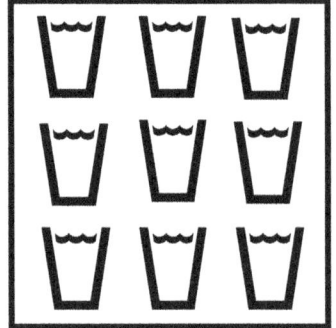

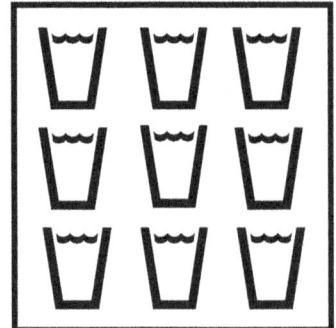

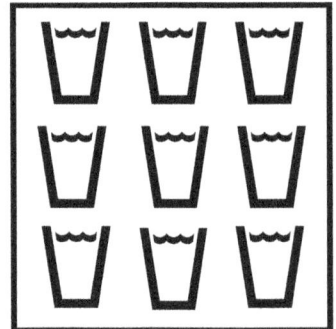

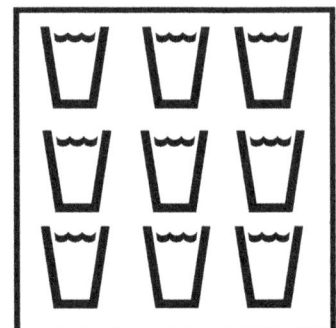

MEAL TRACKER

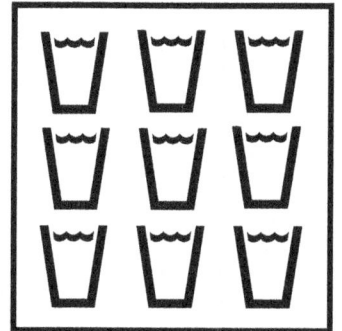

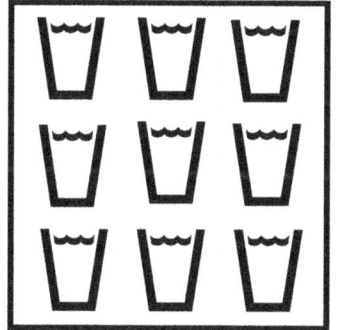

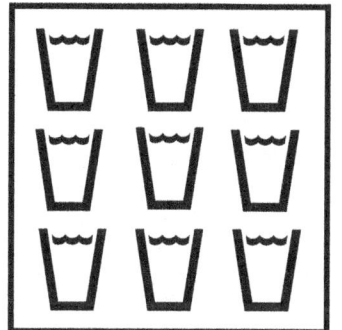

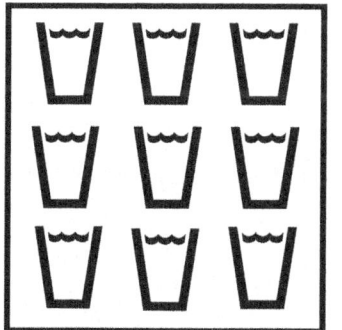

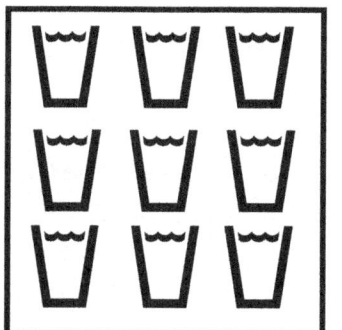

MEAL TRACKER

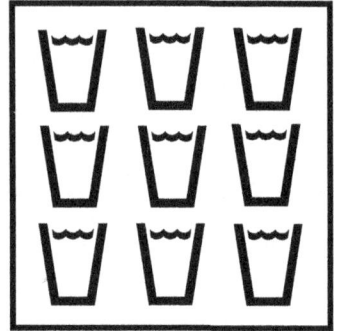

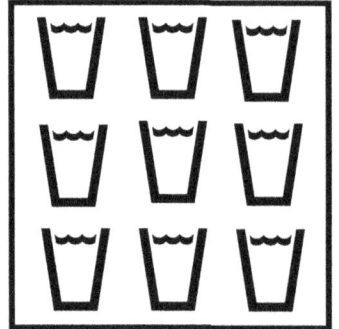

ROUND OVERVIEW

How many times did you eat fast food?

How many times did you cook your own meals?

Did you step out of your comfort zone with any meals?

How was your water intake?

What do you plan to change about your meals next round?

List 3 meals you'd like to cut out.

List 3 new meals you'd like to try.

ROUND OVERVIEW

DID YOU ACCOMPLISH YOUR GOAL WEIGHT? IF YES, WHAT DID YOU REWARD YOURSELF WITH AND WHY?

WERE YOU SUCCESSFUL IN CONTROLLING OR ENDING ANY BAD HABITS? WHICH HABITS DO YOU THINK WILL REQUIRE MORE OF YOUR TIME? DID YOU TAKE ON ANY GOOD HABITS? WHAT WERE THEY? WHAT HABITS ARE YOU INTERESTED IN WORKING ON NEXT ROUND?

HOW WERE YOUR MOODS THIS MONTH? WHAT HAVE YOU DONE FOR YOURSELF? HOW DO YOU FEEL AFTER COMPLETING THIS ROUND?

HOW'D THE SELF CARE REMINDER GO? HOW MANY TIMES DID YOU CATER TO YOURSELF? WHAT DO YOU HAVE PLANNED TO TREAT YOURSELF NEXT ROUND?

DID YOU TRY MEAL PLANNING THIS MONTH? DISCOVER ANY NEW RECIPES OR FOODS YOU ENJOYED? CHOOSE A DAY THAT WOULD BE GOOD FOR YOU TO MEAL PREP FOR THE WEEK.

HOW ACTIVE WERE YOU THIS ROUND? WHAT WAS YOUR MOST FREQUENT ACTIVITY? HOW DO YOU PLAN TO BE MORE ACTIVE NEXT ROUND? ANYTHING NEW YOU'D LIKE TO TRY?

WHAT DID YOUR SLEEP TRACKER REVEAL? HOW HAS IT CHANGED? TRY ANY OF OF THE TIPS/EXERCISES? WHICH ONES WERE HELPFUL?

ROUND 8

GOOD THINGS TAKE TIME.

Stop thinking about what they're thinking about you.
Unknown

GOALS

HABIT TRACKER

Here is where you'll track your habits. In this round the dates are provided so jot down the name of the habit you are working towards or determined to break on the line below. (Ex: Fast food, Exercise, Smoking, etc.) Each day you are successful in either achieving or breaking this habit, you'll highlight or circle the date. The ultimate goal as you continue on through your rounds is to have the whole month colored in. The key is to break bad habits and enforce good ones.

1 2 3 4 5 6 7 8 9
10 11 12 13 14 15 16
17 18 19 20 21 22 23
24 25 26 27 28 29
30 31

_____

1 2 3 4 5 6 7 8 9
10 11 12 13 14 15 16
17 18 19 20 21 22 23
24 25 26 27 28 29
30 31

_____

1 2 3 4 5 6 7 8 9
10 11 12 13 14 15 16
17 18 19 20 21 22 23
24 25 26 27 28 29
30 31

_____

1 2 3 4 5 6 7 8 9
10 11 12 13 14 15 16
17 18 19 20 21 22 23
24 25 26 27 28 29
30 31

_____

MOOD TRACKER

Here is where you'll track your moods daily. Each round you will do this to track how you're feeling throughout your journey. In the "Key" box below, choose your moods and colors to represent them. Each day color in the hearts according to your mood. You're allowed to have good days and bad days. It's perfectly normal throughout your journey. It's called a journey for a reason, you aren't to be in the same place the entire time. Your health, mental state and appearance are all subject to change. Allow yourself to be human and allow yourself the necessary room to grow.

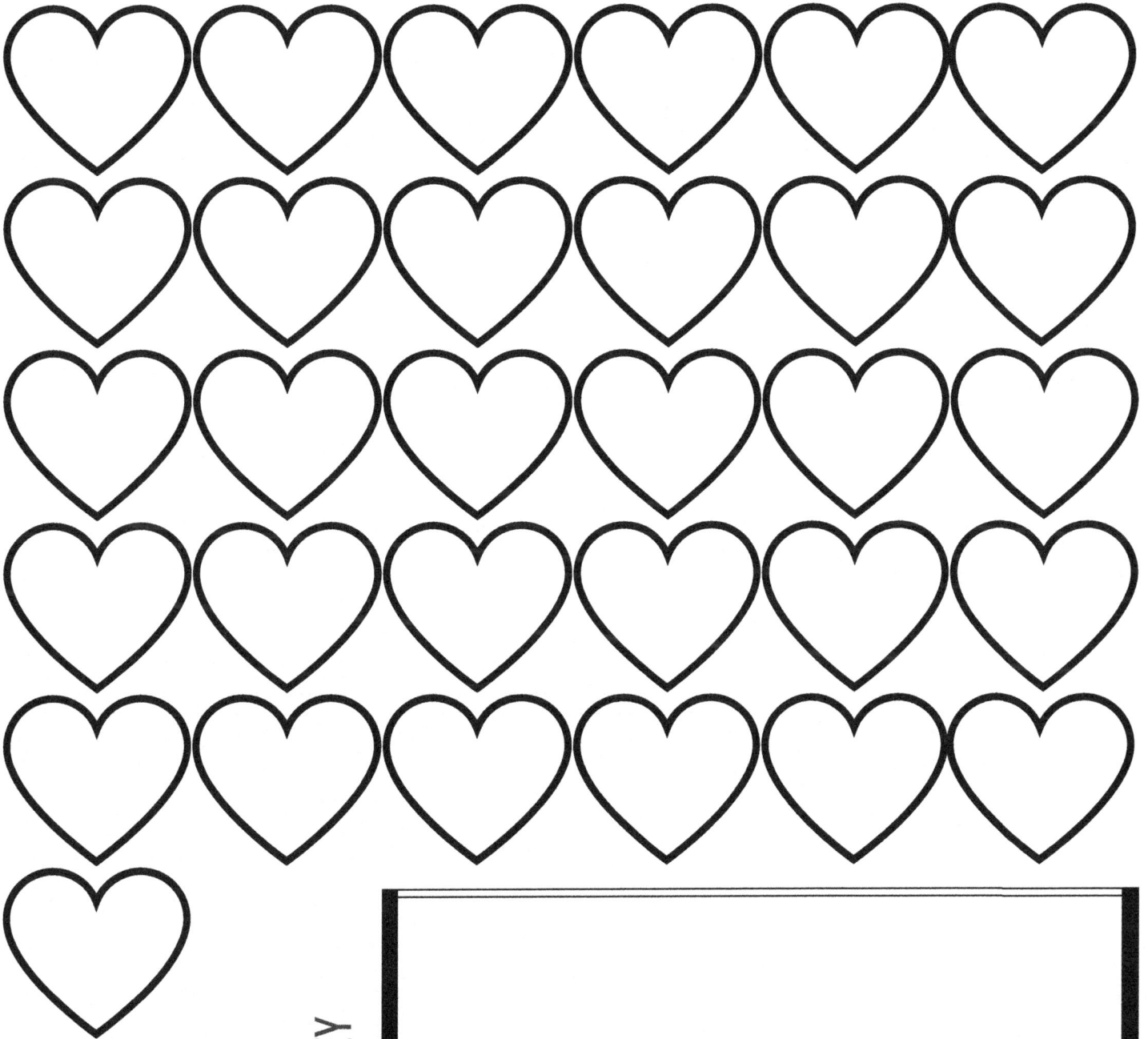

KEY

30 DAYS OF SELF CARE

For this portion you will list 30 acts of self care for each day this month. This is a challenge for you to spend a bit more time taking care of yourself. Be sure to include physical, mental and spiritual acts for the month. Cater to your overall health. When you've completed that task, come back and highlight it.

S	M	T	W	T	F	S

KEY

MENTAL HEALTH CHECK IN

This portion is a free write. Come back here as often as you'd like to pour out your feelings of how your journey is going. Some days are much harder than others and its helpful to get it out your head and jot it down. Just a few minutes a day, take a moment to free your mind here. You'll like to look back on this as well throughout your journey to reflect on your mindset at the start of your journey.

GRATITUDE LOG

This portion is a free write. Come back here as often as you'd like to pour out your feelings of gratitude during this round. You'll like to look back on this as well throughout your journey to reflect on your mindset at the start of your journey.

MONTH OVERVIEW

This undated calendar is for you to track and schedule activities. Anything from work to preferred gym days, meal planning, and even mental health days. Use the "Key" box below to color code all your plans and activities. Think of it as a "YOU" calendar. Everything YOU need to do for yourself to be successful on this journey, plan it all out here.

S	M	T	W	T	F	S

KEY

MEAL PLANNING

This portion is for planning meals ahead. Come back here as often as you'd like to plan your meals or even make grocery lists. You'll like to look back on this as well throughout your journey to reflect on your mindset at the start of your journey.

	S	M	T	W
BREAKFAST				
LUNCH				
DINNER				
SNACKS				

MEAL PLANNING

T	F	S	SHOPPING LIST

SLEEP TRACKER

31
30
29
28
27
26
25
24
23
22
21
20
19
18
17
16
15
14
13
12
11
10
9
8
7
6
5
4
3
2
1

6 7 8 9 10 11 12 1 2 3 4 5 6 7 8 9 10 11 12

WORKOUT LOG

	S	M	T	W	T	F	S
WEEK 1							
WEEK 2							
WEEK 3							
WEEK 4							

KEY

MEAL TRACKER

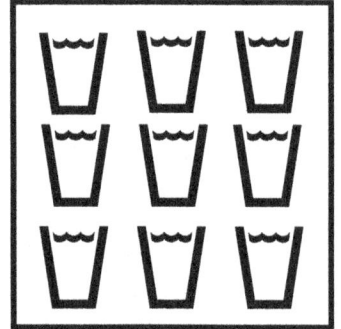

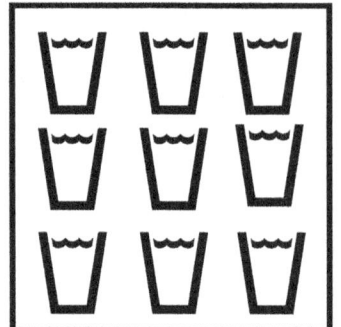

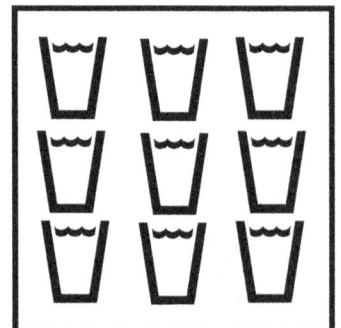

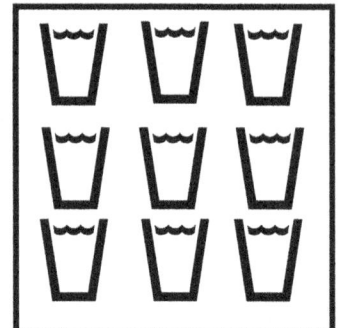

MEAL TRACKER

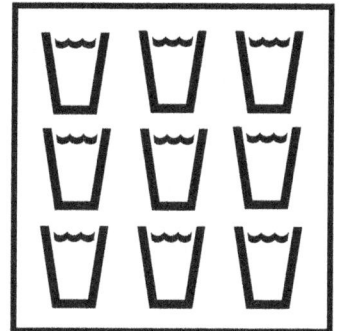

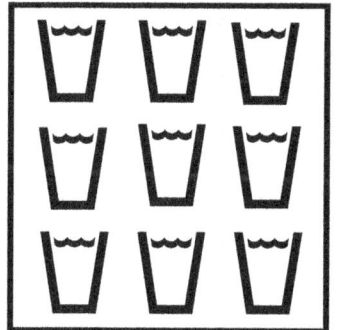

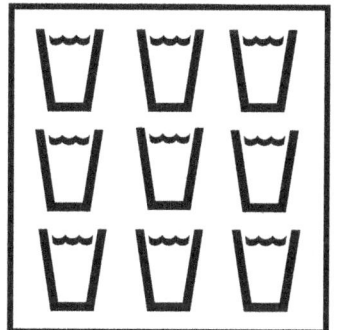

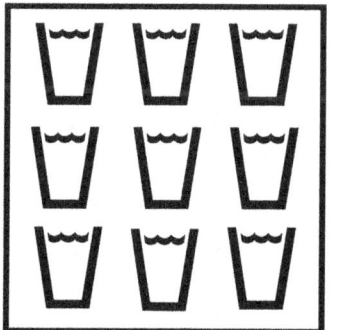

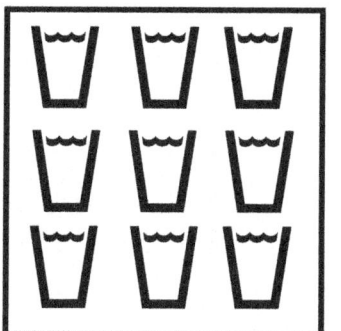

MEAL TRACKER

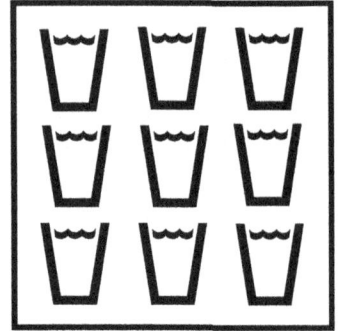

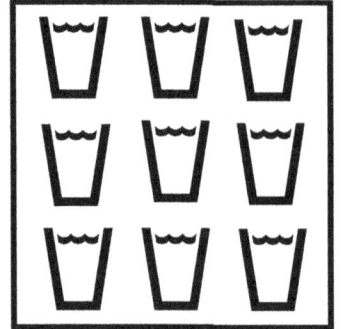

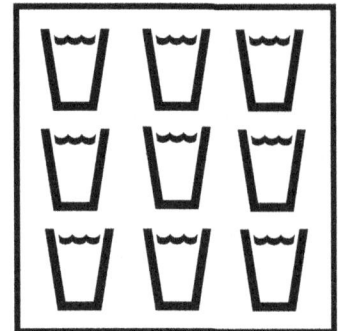

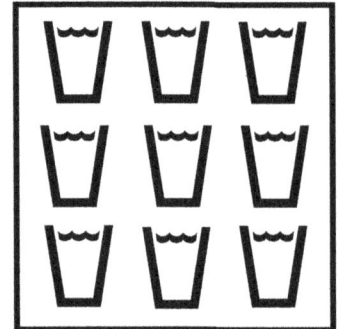

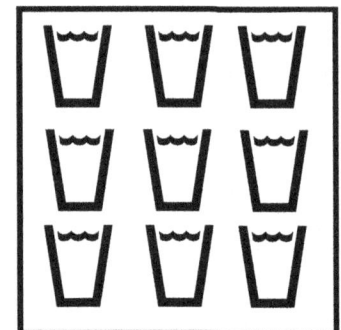

MEAL TRACKER

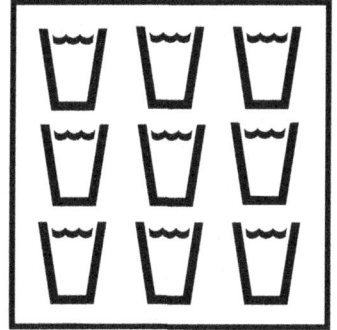

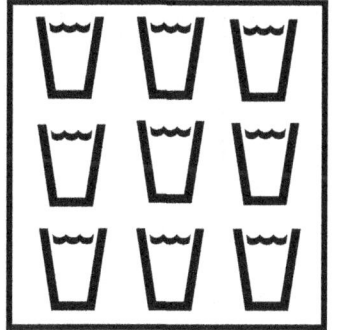

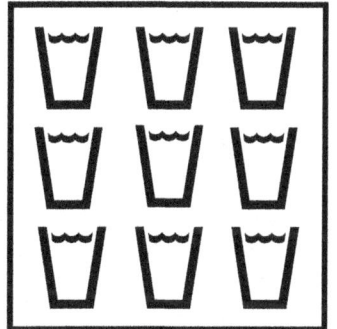

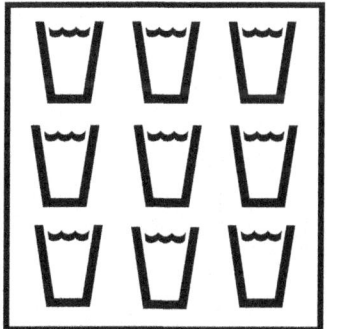

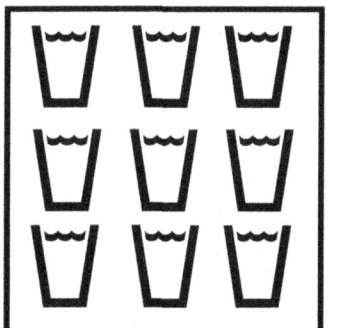

MEAL TRACKER

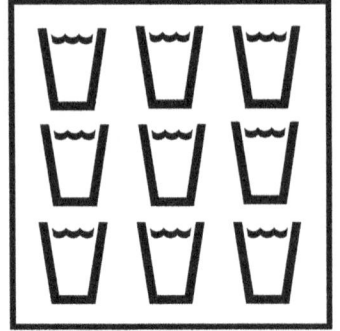

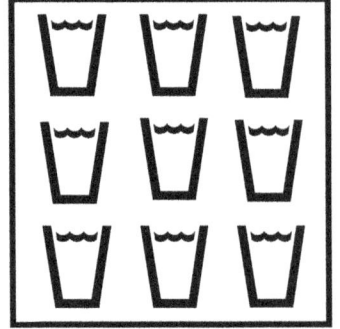

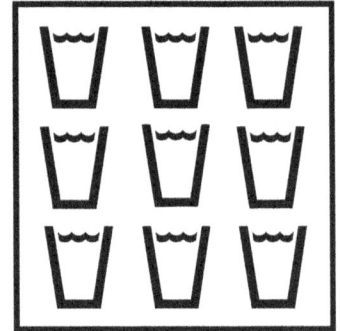

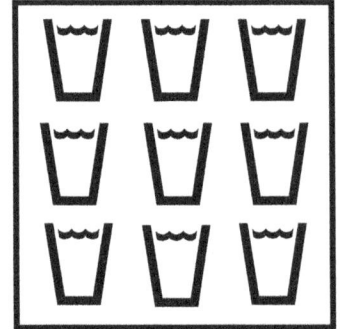

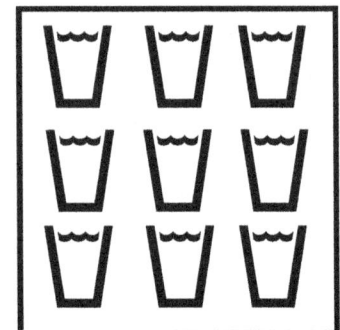

MEAL TRACKER

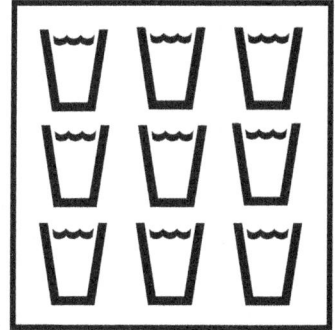

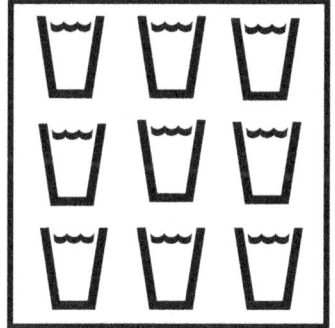

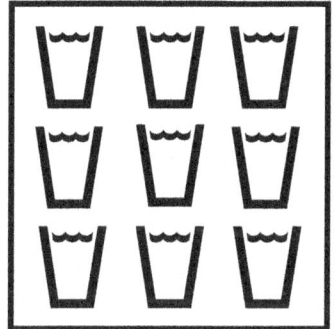

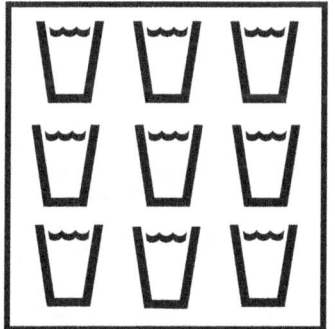

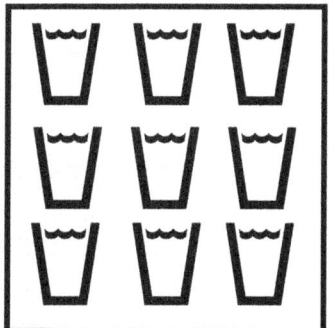

MEAL TRACKER

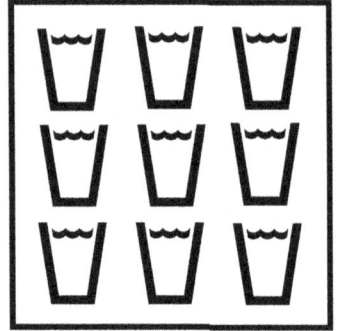

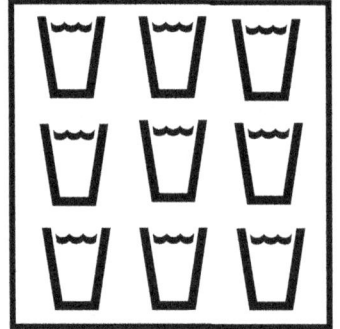

ROUND OVERVIEW

How many times did you eat fast food?

How many times did you cook your own meals?

Did you step out of your comfort zone with any meals?

How was your water intake?

What do you plan to change about your meals next round?

List 3 meals you'd like to cut out.

List 3 new meals you'd like to try.

ROUND OVERVIEW

DID YOU ACCOMPLISH YOUR GOAL WEIGHT? IF YES, WHAT DID YOU REWARD YOURSELF WITH AND WHY?

WERE YOU SUCCESSFUL IN CONTROLLING OR ENDING ANY BAD HABITS? WHICH HABITS DO YOU THINK WILL REQUIRE MORE OF YOUR TIME? DID YOU TAKE ON ANY GOOD HABITS? WHAT WERE THEY? WHAT HABITS ARE YOU INTERESTED IN WORKING ON NEXT ROUND?

HOW WERE YOUR MOODS THIS MONTH? WHAT HAVE YOU DONE FOR YOURSELF? HOW DO YOU FEEL AFTER COMPLETING THIS ROUND?

HOW'D THE SELF CARE REMINDER GO? HOW MANY TIMES DID YOU CATER TO YOURSELF? WHAT DO YOU HAVE PLANNED TO TREAT YOURSELF NEXT ROUND?

DID YOU TRY MEAL PLANNING THIS MONTH? DISCOVER ANY NEW RECIPES OR FOODS YOU ENJOYED? CHOOSE A DAY THAT WOULD BE GOOD FOR YOU TO MEAL PREP FOR THE WEEK.

HOW ACTIVE WERE YOU THIS ROUND? WHAT WAS YOUR MOST FREQUENT ACTIVITY? HOW DO YOU PLAN TO BE MORE ACTIVE NEXT ROUND? ANYTHING NEW YOU'D LIKE TO TRY?

WHAT DID YOUR SLEEP TRACKER REVEAL? HOW HAS IT CHANGED? TRY ANY OF OF THE TIPS/EXERCISES? WHICH ONES WERE HELPFUL?

ROUND 9

GREAT THINGS NEVER CAME FROM
COMFORT ZONES.

The most reliable way
to predict the future is
to create it.
Unknown

Goals

MOOD TRACKER

Here is where you'll track your moods daily. Each round you will do this to track how you're feeling throughout your journey. In the "Key" box below, choose your moods and colors to represent them. Each day color in the hearts according to your mood. You're allowed to have good days and bad days. It's perfectly normal throughout your journey. It's called a journey for a reason, you aren't to be in the same place the entire time. Your health, mental state and appearance are all subject to change. Allow yourself to be human and allow yourself the necessary room to grow.

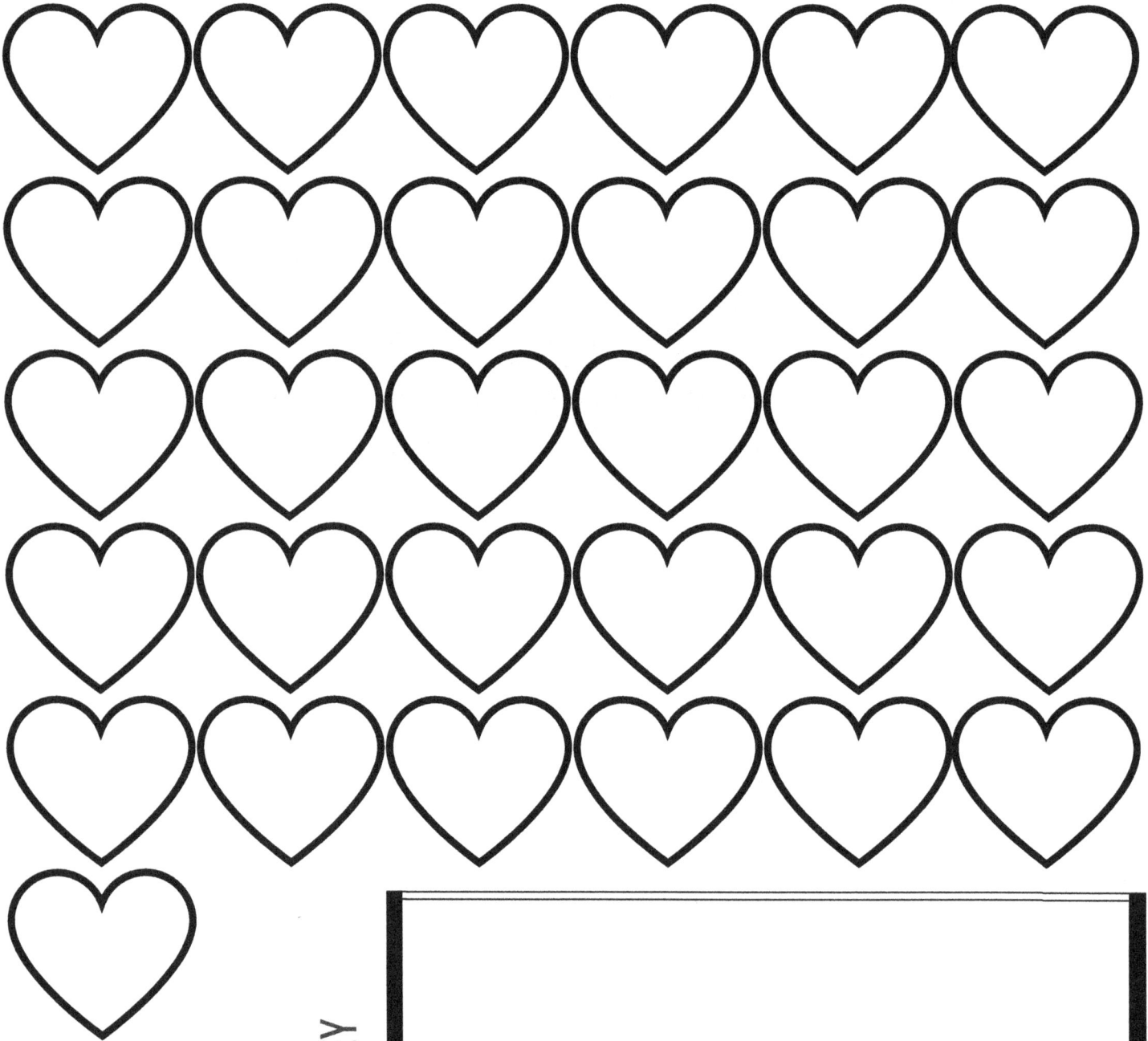

KEY

30 DAYS OF SELF CARE

For this portion you will list 30 acts of self care for each day this month. This is a challenge for you to spend a bit more time taking care of yourself. Be sure to include physical, mental and spiritual acts for the month. Cater to your overall health. When you've completed that task, come back and highlight it.

S	M	T	W	T	F	S

KEY

What Makes Me Happy?

This portion is a little different than the others. Here you will fill this page with ANY and EVERYTHING that makes you happy. This is a reflecting portion.

MENTAL HEALTH CHECK IN

This portion is a free write. Come back here as often as you'd like to pour out your feelings of how your journey is going. Some days are much harder than others and its helpful to get it out your head and jot it down. Just a few minutes a day, take a moment to free your mind here. You'll like to look back on this as well throughout your journey to reflect on your mindset at the start of your journey.

GRATITUDE LOG

This portion is a free write. Come back here as often as you'd like to pour out your feelings of gratitude during this round. You'll like to look back on this as well throughout your journey to reflect on your mindset at the start of your journey.

PROGRESS TRACKER

This portion is a mid journey reflection how how many pounds you've lost/gained so far on this journey & how much closer you are to your goal! List the date your journey began, as well as your starting weight and goal weight! Then draw circles or hearts in the bottom jar, representing how many pounds you've already lost/gained and do the same in the top jar representing how many more pounds are left to reach your goal weight for this journey!

Start Date:

Starting Weight:

Goal Weight:

HOW MANY TO GO

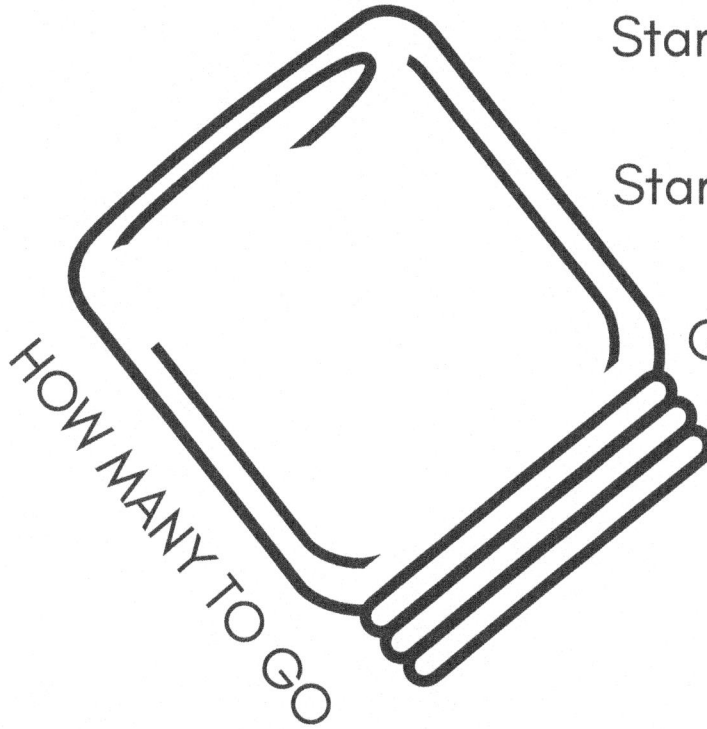

LITTLE by LITTLE, a LITTLE becomes a **LOT**

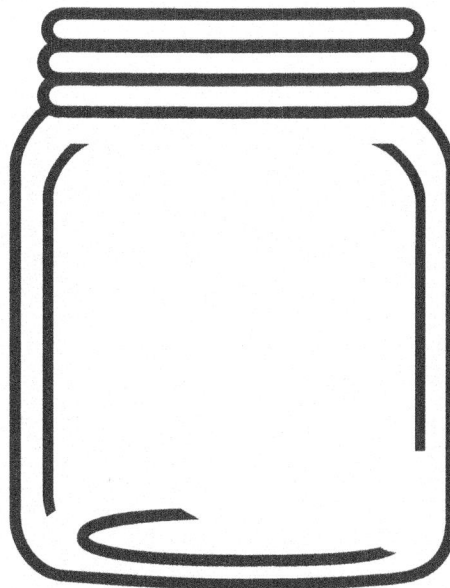

HOW MANY LOST/GAINED

SLEEP TRACKER

31
30
29
28
27
26
25
24
23
22
21
20
19
18
17
16
15
14
13
12
11
10
9
8
7
6
5
4
3
2
1

6   7   8   9   10   11   12   1   2   3   4   5   6   7   8   9   10   11   12

WORKOUT LOG

	S	M	T	W	T	F	S
WEEK 1							
WEEK 2							
WEEK 3							
WEEK 4							

KEY

MEAL TRACKER

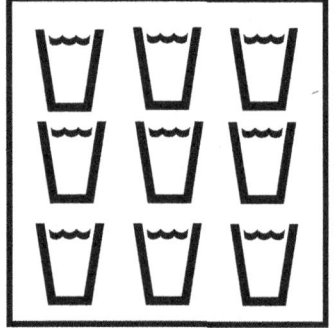

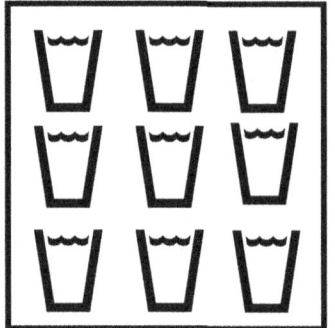

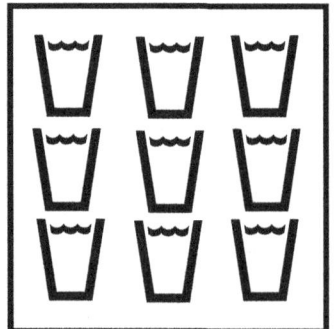

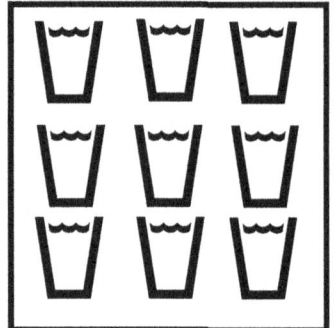

MEAL TRACKER

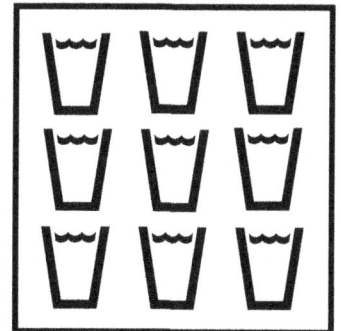

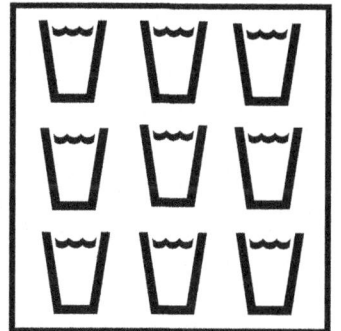

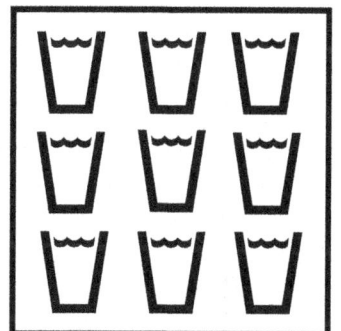

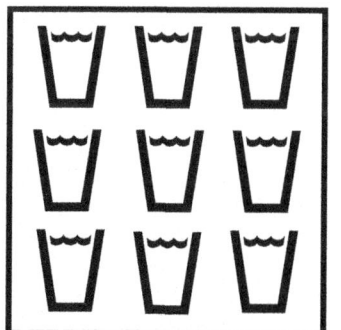

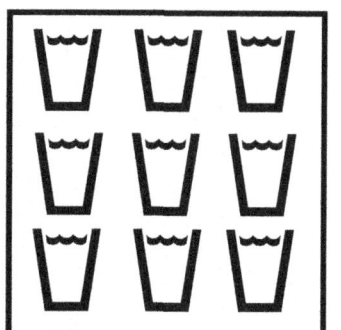

MEAL TRACKER

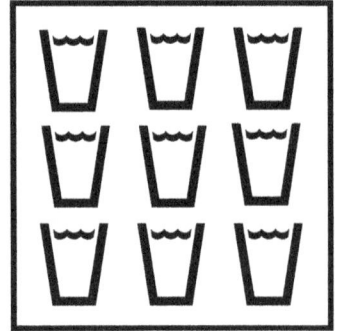

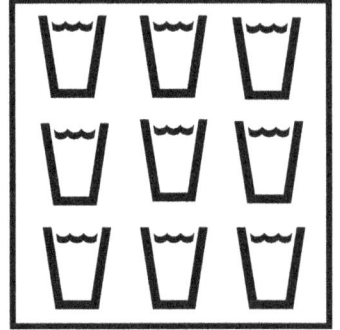

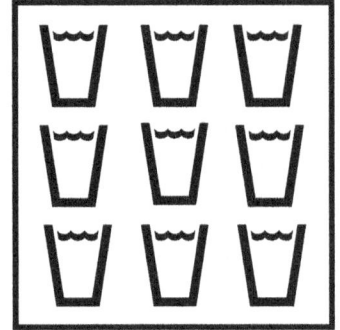

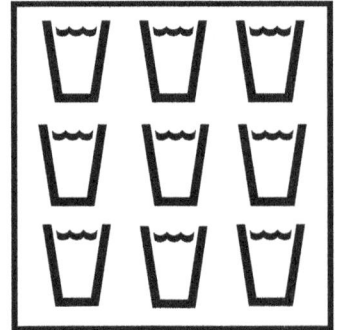

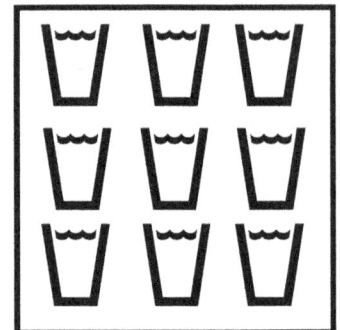

MEAL TRACKER

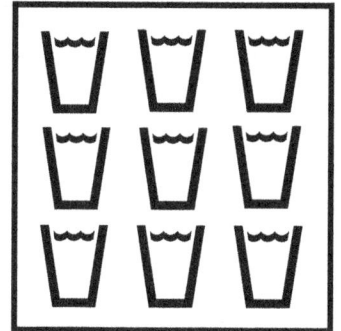

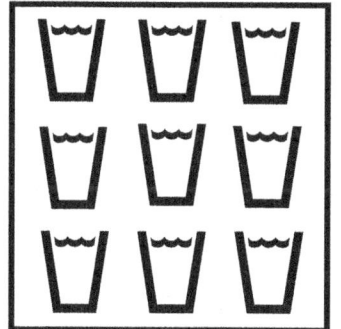

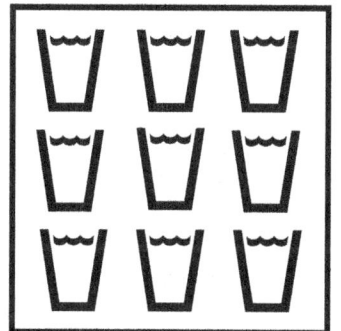

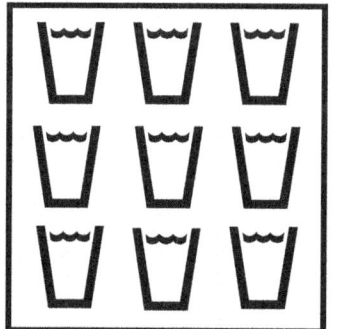

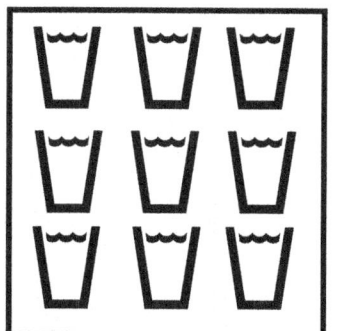

MEAL TRACKER

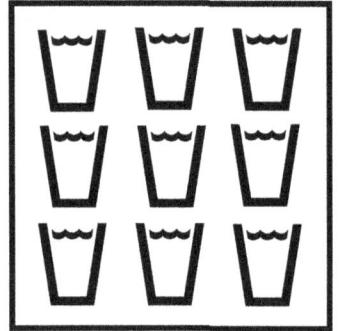

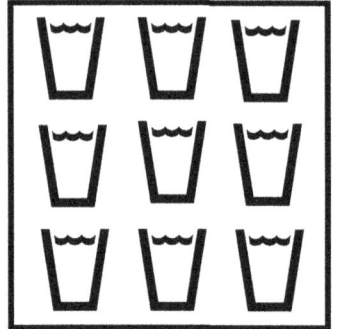

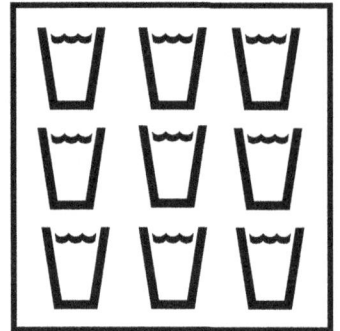

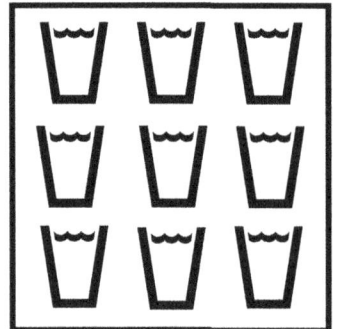

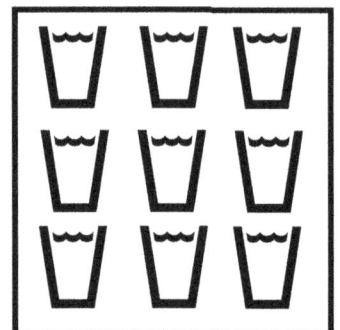

MEAL TRACKER

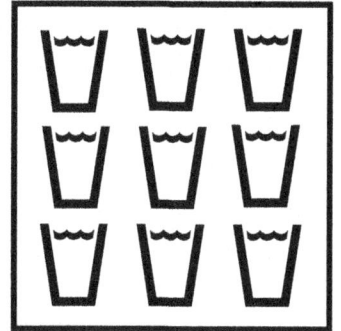

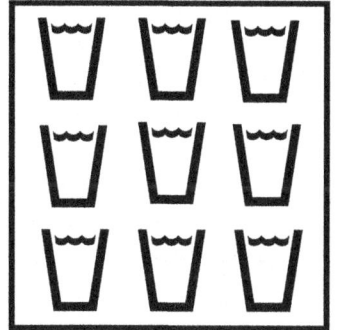

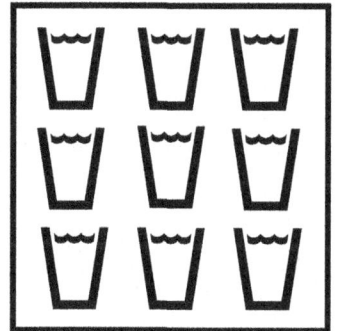

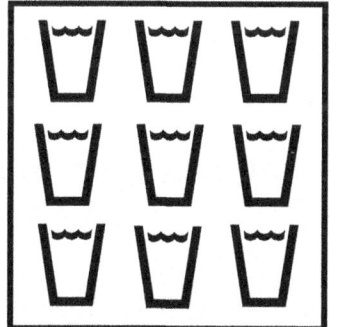

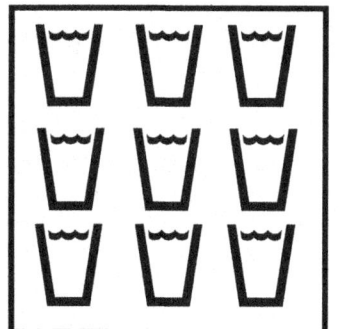

MEAL TRACKER

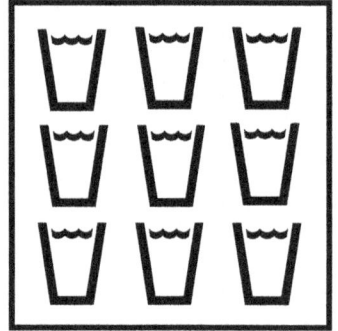

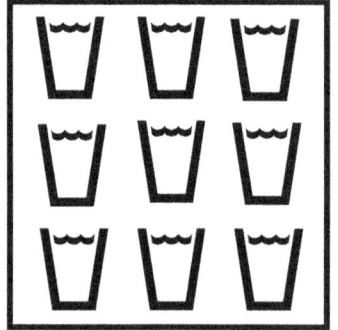

ROUND OVERVIEW

How many times did you eat fast food?

How many times did you cook your own meals?

Did you step out of your comfort zone with any meals?

How was your water intake?

What do you plan to change about your meals next round?

List 3 meals you'd like to cut out.

List 3 new meals you'd like to try.

ROUND OVERVIEW

DID YOU ACCOMPLISH YOUR GOAL WEIGHT? IF YES, WHAT DID YOU REWARD YOURSELF WITH AND WHY?

WERE YOU SUCCESSFUL IN CONTROLLING OR ENDING ANY BAD HABITS? WHICH HABITS DO YOU THINK WILL REQUIRE MORE OF YOUR TIME? DID YOU TAKE ON ANY GOOD HABITS? WHAT WERE THEY? WHAT HABITS ARE YOU INTERESTED IN WORKING ON NEXT ROUND?

HOW WERE YOUR MOODS THIS MONTH? WHAT HAVE YOU DONE FOR YOURSELF? HOW DO YOU FEEL AFTER COMPLETING THIS ROUND?

HOW'D THE SELF CARE REMINDER GO? HOW MANY TIMES DID YOU CATER TO YOURSELF? WHAT DO YOU HAVE PLANNED TO TREAT YOURSELF NEXT ROUND?

DID YOU TRY MEAL PLANNING THIS MONTH? DISCOVER ANY NEW RECIPES OR FOODS YOU ENJOYED? CHOOSE A DAY THAT WOULD BE GOOD FOR YOU TO MEAL PREP FOR THE WEEK.

HOW ACTIVE WERE YOU THIS ROUND? WHAT WAS YOUR MOST FREQUENT ACTIVITY? HOW DO YOU PLAN TO BE MORE ACTIVE NEXT ROUND? ANYTHING NEW YOU'D LIKE TO TRY?

WHAT DID YOUR SLEEP TRACKER REVEAL? HOW HAS IT CHANGED? TRY ANY OF OF THE TIPS/EXERCISES? WHICH ONES WERE HELPFUL?

JOURNEY REFLECTIONS

WHAT GOALS ARE YOU MOST PROUD OF ACCOMPLISHING SINCE STARTING YOUR JOURNEY?

REFLECTING ON BAD HABITS FROM ROUND 1, WHAT HABITS HAVE YOU ELIMINATED AND GAINED DURING THIS JOURNEY?

HOW HAVE YOUR MOODS BEEN OVER THE LAST 9 ROUNDS? DO YOU NOTICE IMPROVEMENTS? HAVE YOU BEEN DOING MORE ACTIVITIES & SPENDING TIME WITH THOSE WHO BRING YOU HAPPINESS?

HOW HELPFUL HAS THE MENTAL CHECK IN BEEN? DO YOU LOG FREQUENTLY?

HOW HELPFUL HAS THE GRATITUDE LOG BEEN? DO YOU LOG FREQUENTLY?

JOURNEY REFLECTIONS

CAN YOU SAY OVER THESE PAST 9 ROUNDS THAT YOU'VE MADE SELF CARE A PART OF YOUR ROUTINE? HOW OFTEN A WEEK ARE YOU SETTING TIME ASIDE TO PRACTICE SELF CARE?

HOW OFTEN HAVE YOU BEEN ACTIVE OVER THESE PAST 9 ROUNDS? HAVE YOU MADE BEING ACTIVE A PART OF YOUR ROUTINE? HOW DOES IT FEEL?

HOW HELPFUL HAS YOUR MANTRA BEEN? DO YOU RECITE IT DAILY? DO YOU HAVE IT MEMORIZED YET?

LIST A FEW WORDS OF ENCOURAGEMENT FOR YOURSELF DURING THE REMAINDER OF YOUR JOURNEY.

ROUND 10

I WILL ALWAYS BE ENOUGH.

Be happy with what you have while working for what you want.
Helen Keller

GETTING TO KNOW YOU

This portion is for you to get to know yourself a little better before we start the first round of your journey. You will do these every 3 rounds. It's a reflection that you'll be happy to look back on at the end of your yearlong journey. Write a short letter to yourself explaining who you are at this point in your life and what has inspired you to embark on this journey. Be honest with yourself. No one will read this but you. Don't overthink it. Just write freely.

GOALS

HABIT TRACKER

Here is where you'll track your habits. In this round the dates are provided so jot down the name of the habit you are working towards or determined to break on the line below. (Ex: Fast food, Exercise, Smoking, etc.) Each day you are successful in either achieving or breaking this habit, you'll highlight or circle the date. The ultimate goal as you continue on through your rounds is to have the whole month colored in. The key is to break bad habits and enforce good ones.

1 2 3 4 5 6 7 8 9
10 11 12 13 14 15 16
17 18 19 20 21 22 23
24 25 26 27 28 29
30 31

_____

1 2 3 4 5 6 7 8 9
10 11 12 13 14 15 16
17 18 19 20 21 22 23
24 25 26 27 28 29
30 31

_____

1 2 3 4 5 6 7 8 9
10 11 12 13 14 15 16
17 18 19 20 21 22 23
24 25 26 27 28 29
30 31

_____

1 2 3 4 5 6 7 8 9
10 11 12 13 14 15 16
17 18 19 20 21 22 23
24 25 26 27 28 29
30 31

_____

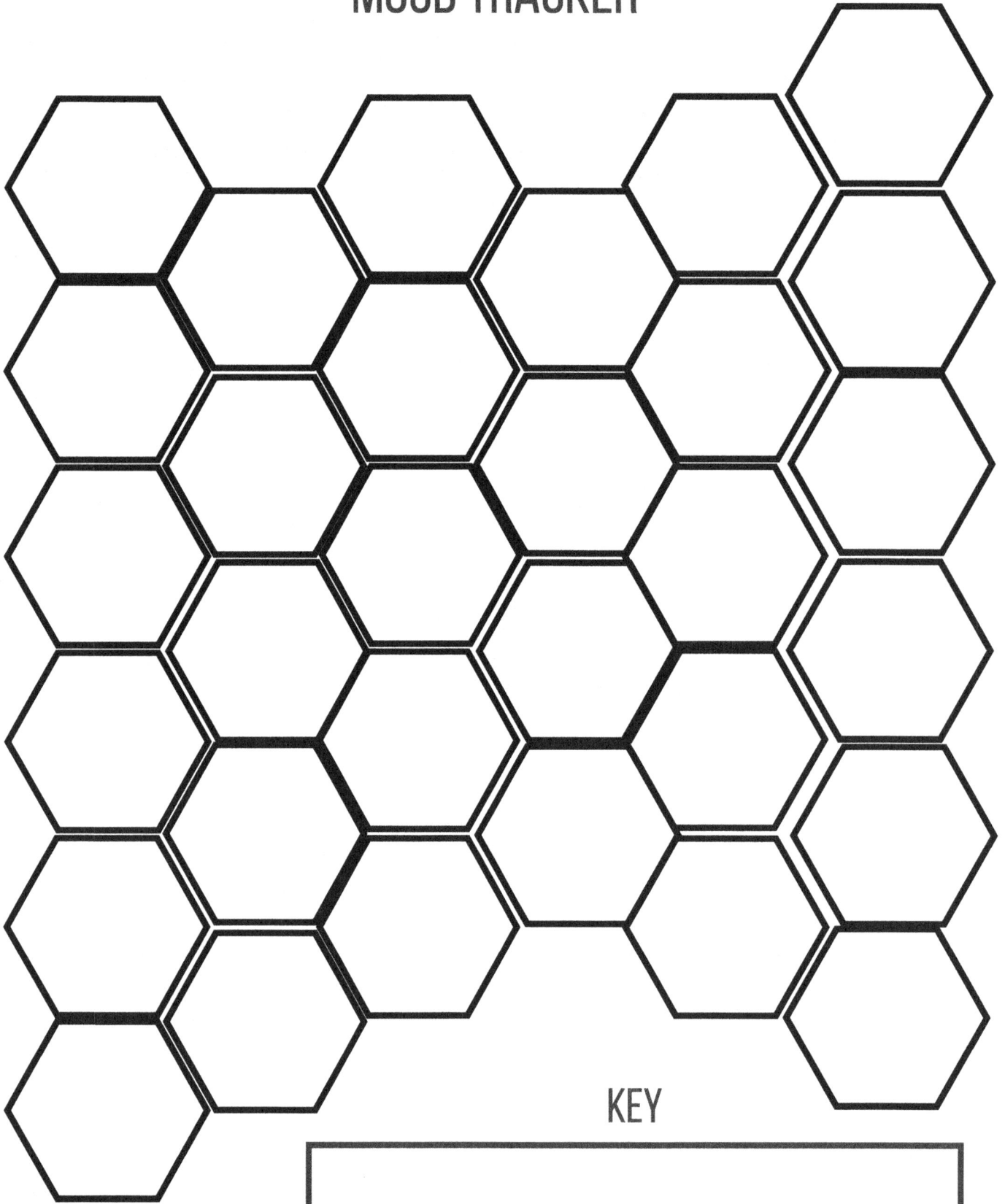

MOOD TRACKER

KEY

30 DAYS OF SELF CARE

For this portion you will list 30 acts of self care for each day this month. This is a challenge for you to spend a bit more time taking care of yourself. Be sure to include physical, mental and spiritual acts for the month. Cater to your overall health. When you've completed that task, come back and highlight it.

S	M	T	W	T	F	S

KEY

MENTAL HEALTH CHECK IN

This portion is a free write. Come back here as often as you'd like to pour out your feelings of how your journey is going. Some days are much harder than others and its helpful to get it out your head and jot it down. Just a few minutes a day, take a moment to free your mind here. You'll like to look back on this as well throughout your journey to reflect on your mindset at the start of your journey.

GRATITUDE LOG

This portion is a free write. Come back here as often as you'd like to pour out your feelings of gratitude during this round. You'll like to look back on this as well throughout your journey to reflect on your mindset at the start of your journey.

MONTH OVERVIEW

This undated calendar is for you to track and schedule activities.Anything from work to preferred gym days, meal planning, and even mental health days. Use the "Key" box below to color code all your plans and activities. Think of it as a "YOU" calendar. Everything YOU need to do for yourself to be successful on this journey, plan it all out here.

S	M	T	W	T	F	S

KEY

MEAL PLANNING

This portion is for planning meals ahead. Come back here as often as you'd like to plan your meals or even make grocery lists. You'll like to look back on this as well throughout your journey to reflect on your mindset at the start of your journey.

	S	M	T	W
BREAKFAST				
LUNCH				
DINNER				
SNACKS				

MEAL PLANNING

T	F	S	SHOPPING LIST

SLEEP TRACKER

31
30
29
28
27
26
25
24
23
22
21
20
19
18
17
16
15
14
13
12
11
10
9
8
7
6
5
4
3
2
1

6 7 8 9 10 11 12 1 2 3 4 5 6 7 8 9 10 11 12

WORKOUT LOG

	S	M	T	W	T	F	S
WEEK 1							
WEEK 2							
WEEK 3							
WEEK 4							

KEY

MEAL TRACKER

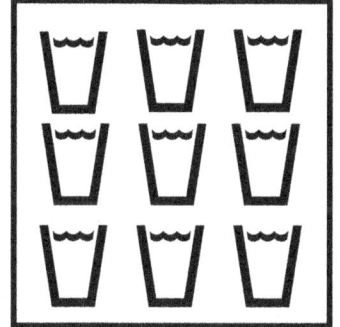

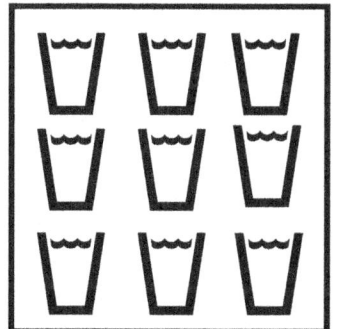

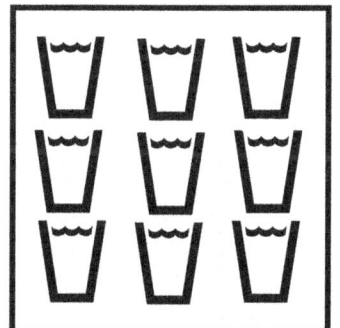

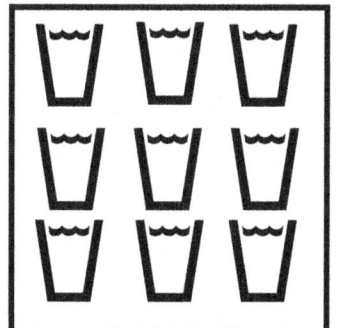

MEAL TRACKER

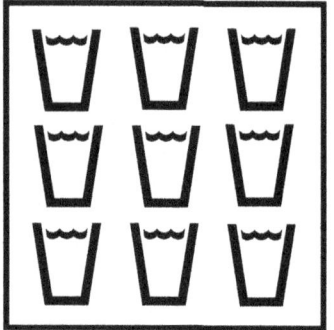

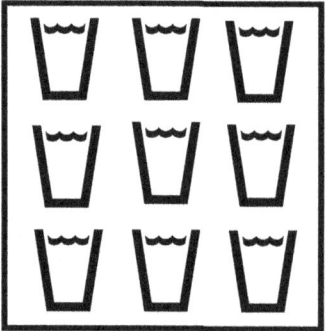

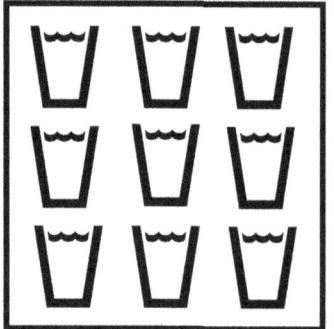

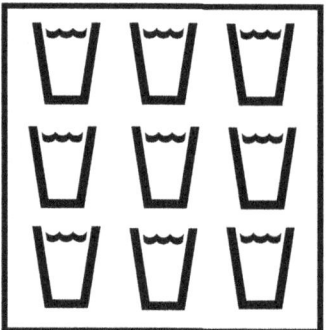

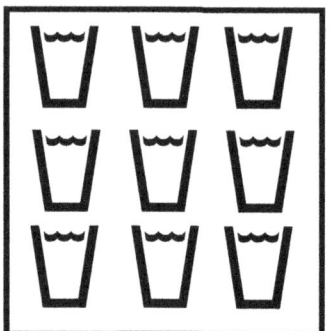

MEAL TRACKER

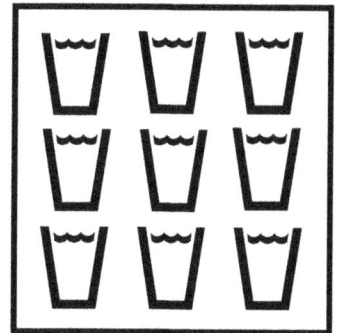

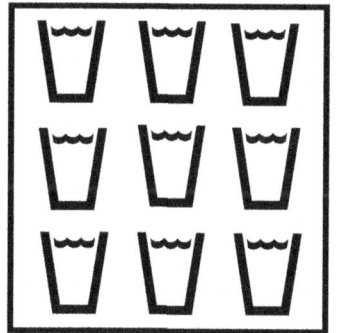

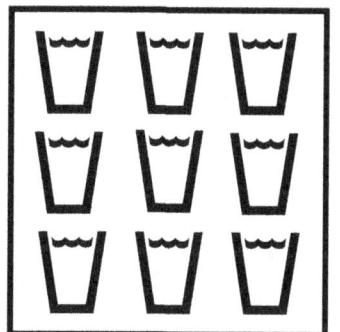

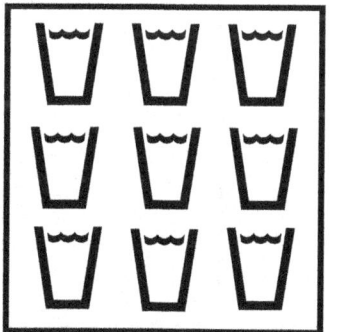

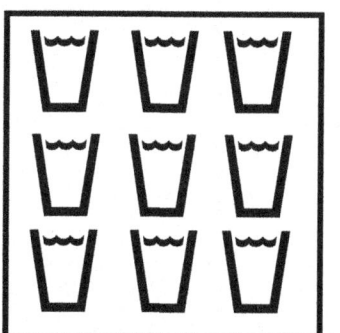

MEAL TRACKER

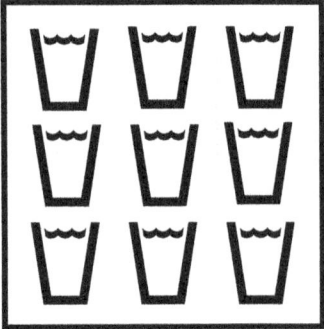

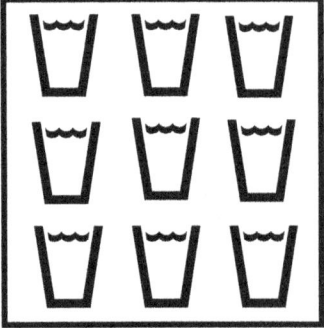

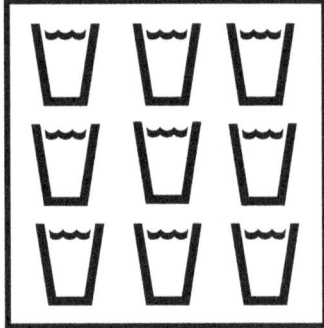

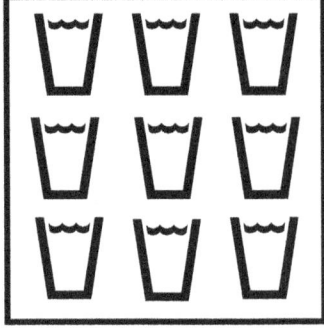

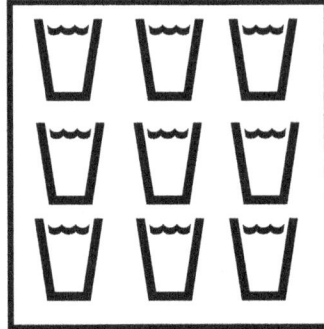

MEAL TRACKER

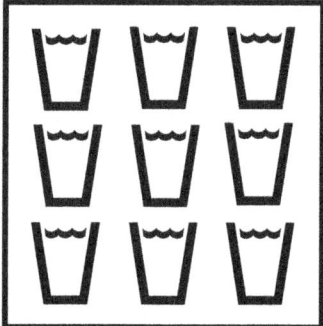

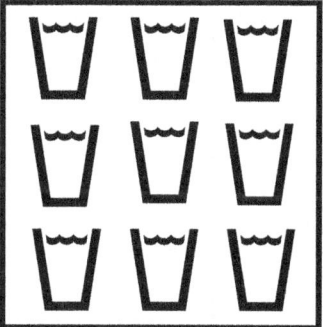

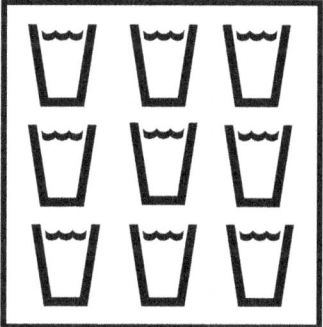

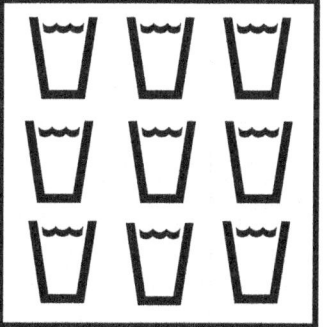

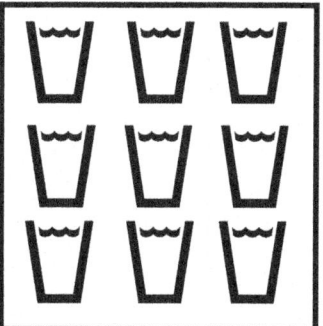

MEAL TRACKER

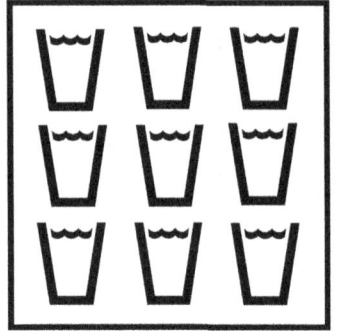

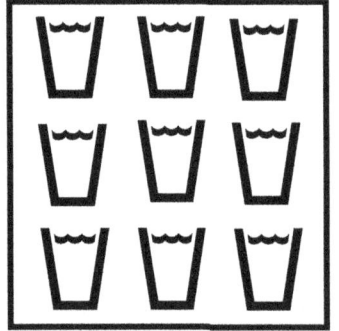

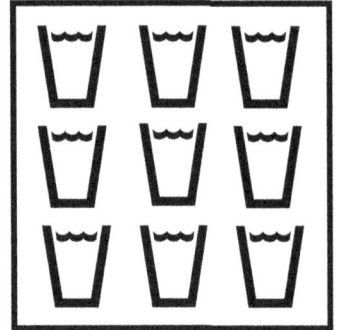

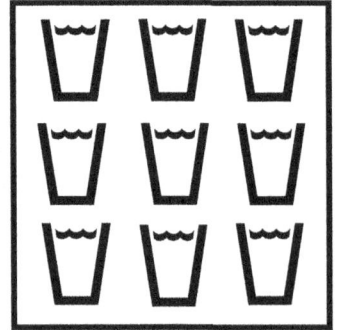

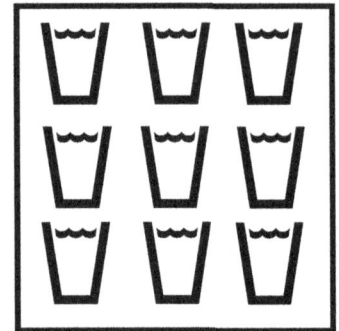

MEAL TRACKER

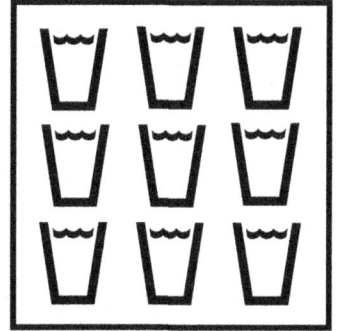

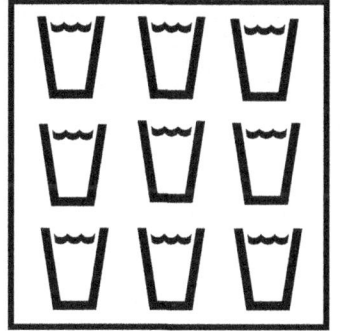

ROUND OVERVIEW

How many times did you eat fast food?

How many times did you cook your own meals?

Did you step out of your comfort zone with any meals?

How was your water intake?

What do you plan to change about your meals next round?

List 3 meals you'd like to cut out.

List 3 new meals you'd like to try.

ROUND OVERVIEW

DID YOU ACCOMPLISH YOUR GOAL WEIGHT? IF YES, WHAT DID YOU REWARD YOURSELF WITH AND WHY?

WERE YOU SUCCESSFUL IN CONTROLLING OR ENDING ANY BAD HABITS? WHICH HABITS DO YOU THINK WILL REQUIRE MORE OF YOUR TIME? DID YOU TAKE ON ANY GOOD HABITS? WHAT WERE THEY? WHAT HABITS ARE YOU INTERESTED IN WORKING ON NEXT ROUND?

HOW WERE YOUR MOODS THIS MONTH? WHAT HAVE YOU DONE FOR YOURSELF? HOW DO YOU FEEL AFTER COMPLETING THIS ROUND?

HOW'D THE SELF CARE REMINDER GO? HOW MANY TIMES DID YOU CATER TO YOURSELF? WHAT DO YOU HAVE PLANNED TO TREAT YOURSELF NEXT ROUND?

DID YOU TRY MEAL PLANNING THIS MONTH? DISCOVER ANY NEW RECIPES OR FOODS YOU ENJOYED? CHOOSE A DAY THAT WOULD BE GOOD FOR YOU TO MEAL PREP FOR THE WEEK.

HOW ACTIVE WERE YOU THIS ROUND? WHAT WAS YOUR MOST FREQUENT ACTIVITY? HOW DO YOU PLAN TO BE MORE ACTIVE NEXT ROUND? ANYTHING NEW YOU'D LIKE TO TRY?

WHAT DID YOUR SLEEP TRACKER REVEAL? HOW HAS IT CHANGED? TRY ANY OF OF THE TIPS/EXERCISES? WHICH ONES WERE HELPFUL?

ROUND 11

REMEMBER WHY YOU STARTED.

I already know what giving up feels like. I want to see what happens if I don't.
Neila Rey

GOALS

HABIT TRACKER

Here is where you'll track your habits. In this round the dates are provided so jot down the name of the habit you are working towards or determined to break on the line below. (Ex: Fast food, Exercise, Smoking, etc.) Each day you are successful in either achieving or breaking this habit, you'll highlight or circle the date. The ultimate goal as you continue on through your rounds is to have the whole month colored in. The key is to break bad habits and enforce good ones.

1 2 3 4 5 6 7 8 9
10 11 12 13 14 15 16
17 18 19 20 21 22 23
24 25 26 27 28 29
30 31

_____

1 2 3 4 5 6 7 8 9
10 11 12 13 14 15 16
17 18 19 20 21 22 23
24 25 26 27 28 29
30 31

_____

1 2 3 4 5 6 7 8 9
10 11 12 13 14 15 16
17 18 19 20 21 22 23
24 25 26 27 28 29
30 31

_____

1 2 3 4 5 6 7 8 9
10 11 12 13 14 15 16
17 18 19 20 21 22 23
24 25 26 27 28 29
30 31

_____

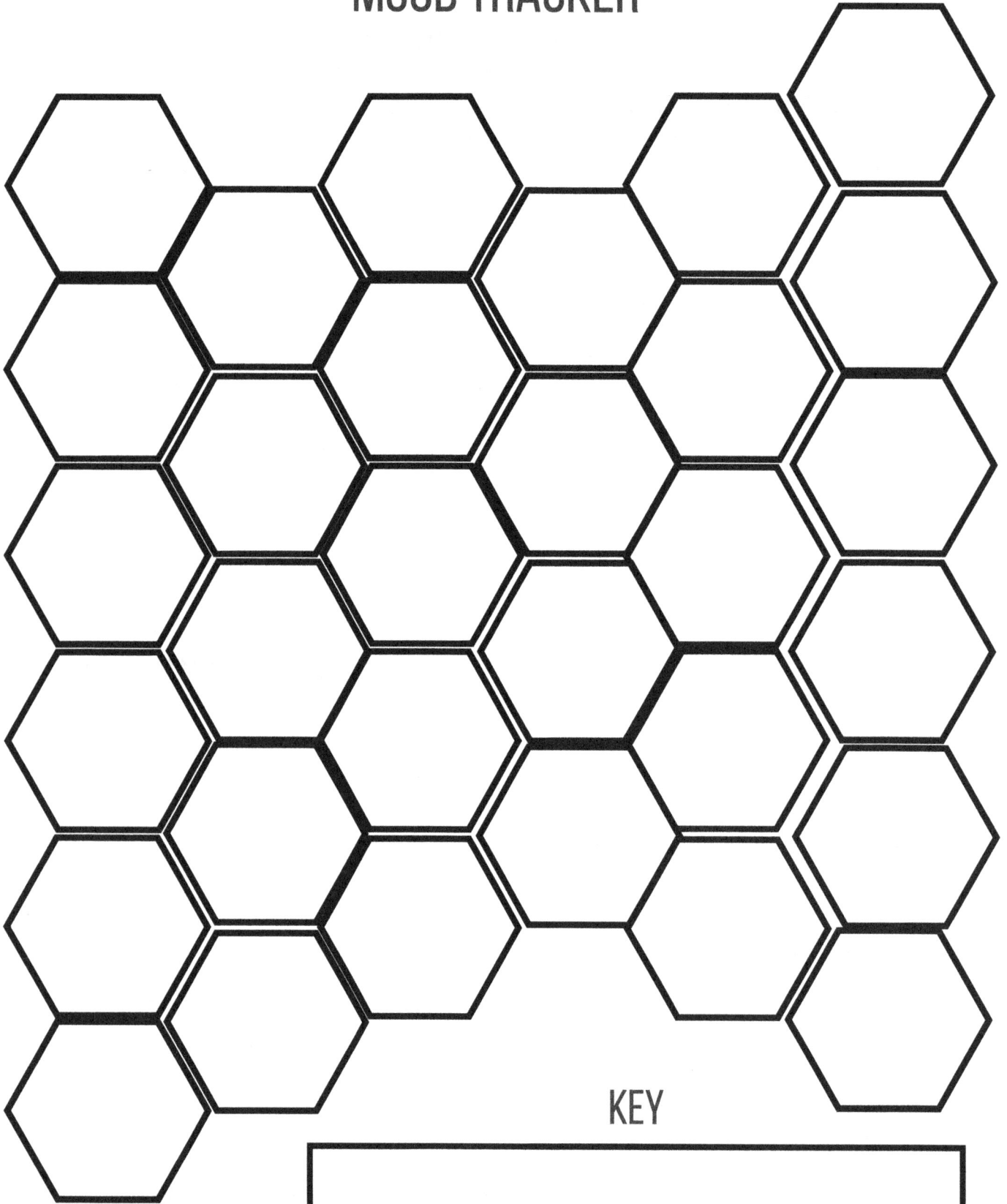

MOOD TRACKER

KEY

30 DAYS OF SELF CARE

For this portion you will list 30 acts of self care for each day this month. This is a challenge for you to spend a bit more time taking care of yourself. Be sure to include physical, mental and spiritual acts for the month. Cater to your overall health. When you've completed that task, come back and highlight it.

S	M	T	W	T	F	S

KEY

MENTAL HEALTH CHECK IN

This portion is a free write. Come back here as often as you'd like to pour out your feelings of how your journey is going. Some days are much harder than others and its helpful to get it out your head and jot it down. Just a few minutes a day, take a moment to free your mind here. You'll like to look back on this as well throughout your journey to reflect on your mindset at the start of your journey.

GRATITUDE LOG

This portion is a free write. Come back here as often as you'd like to pour out your feelings of gratitude during this round. You'll like to look back on this as well throughout your journey to reflect on your mindset at the start of your journey.

MONTH OVERVIEW

This undated calendar is for you to track and schedule activities. Anything from work to preferred gym days, meal planning, and even mental health days. Use the "Key" box below to color code all your plans and activities. Think of it as a "YOU" calendar. Everything YOU need to do for yourself to be successful on this journey, plan it all out here.

S	M	T	W	T	F	S

KEY

MEAL PLANNING

This portion is for planning meals ahead. Come back here as often as you'd like to plan your meals or even make grocery lists. You'll like to look back on this as well throughout your journey to reflect on your mindset at the start of your journey.

	S	M	T	W
BREAKFAST				
LUNCH				
DINNER				
SNACKS				

MEAL PLANNING

T	F	S	SHOPPING LIST

SLEEP TRACKER

31
30
29
28
27
26
25
24
23
22
21
20
19
18
17
16
15
14
13
12
11
10
9
8
7
6
5
4
3
2
1

6 7 8 9 10 11 12 1 2 3 4 5 6 7 8 9 10 11 12

WORKOUT LOG

	S	M	T	W	T	F	S
WEEK 1							
WEEK 2							
WEEK 3							
WEEK 4							

KEY

MEAL TRACKER

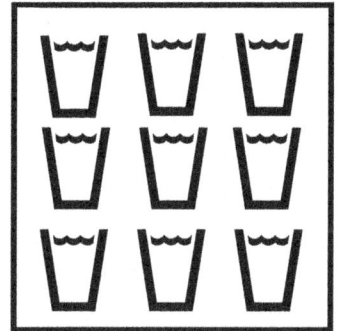

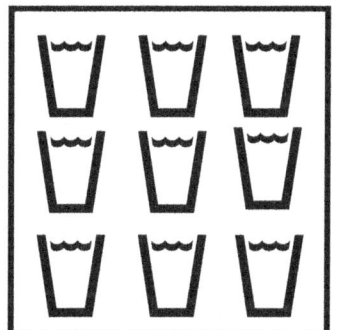

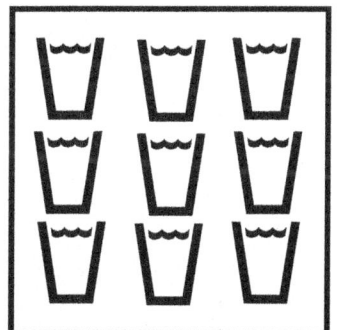

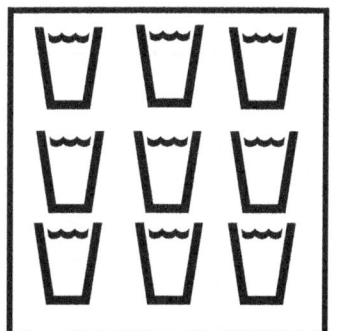

MEAL TRACKER

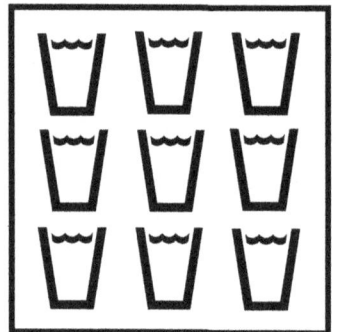

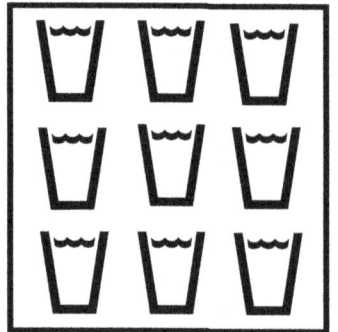

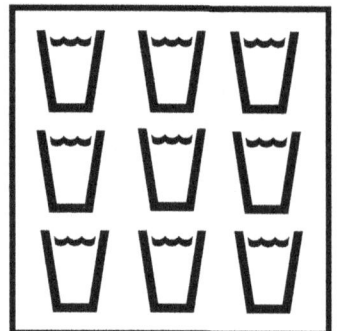

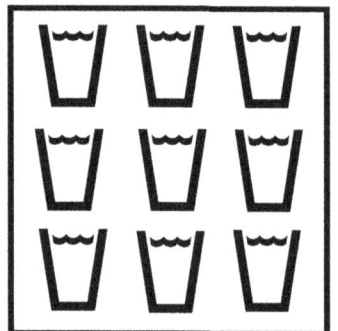

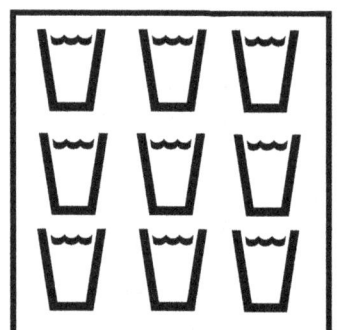

MEAL TRACKER

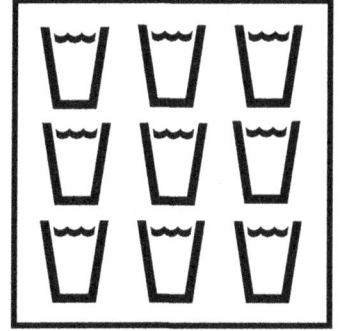

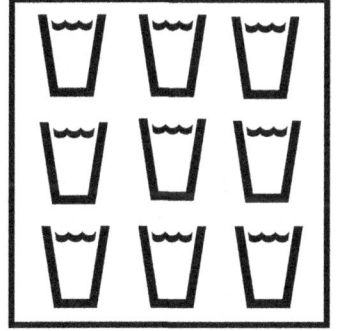

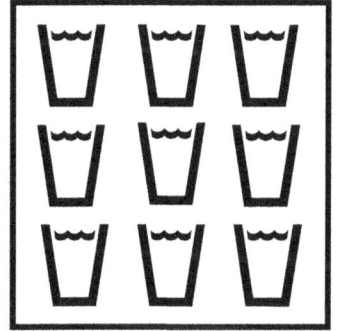

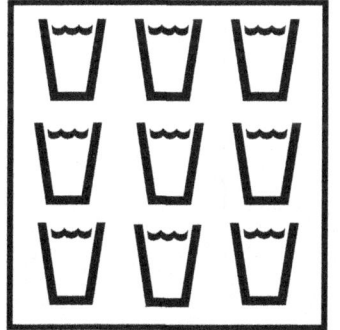

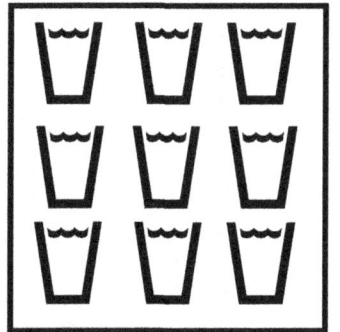

MEAL TRACKER

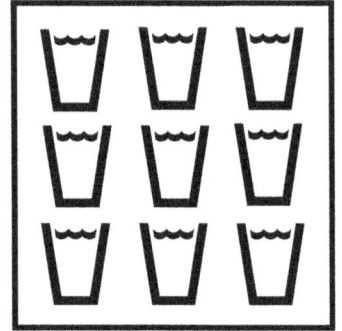

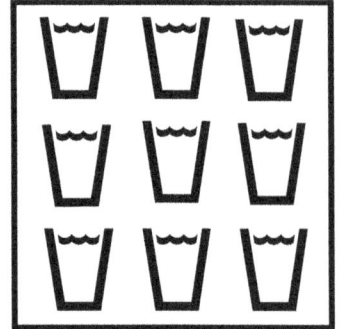

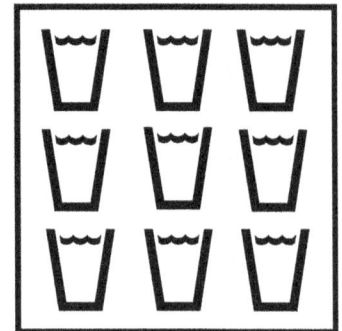

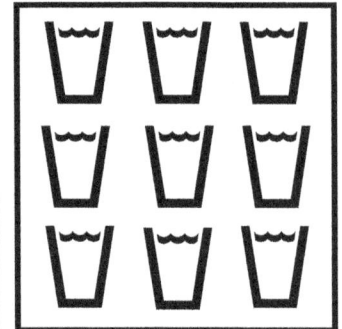

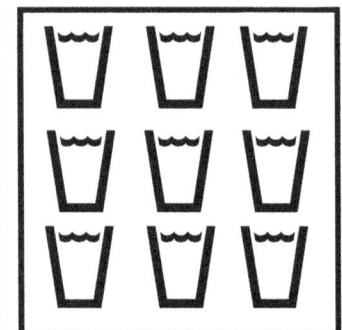

MEAL TRACKER

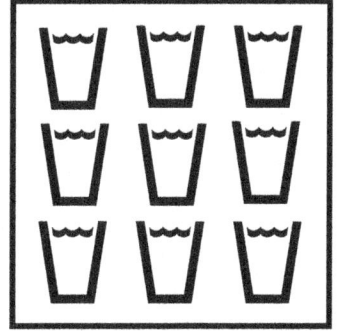

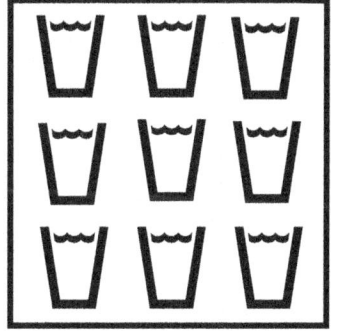

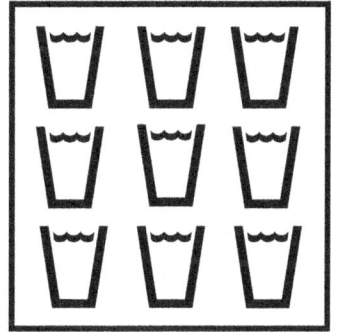

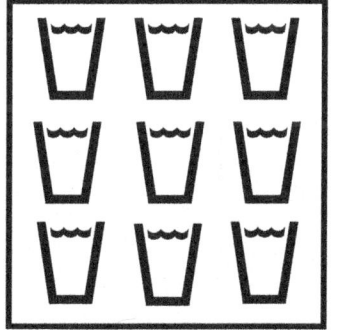

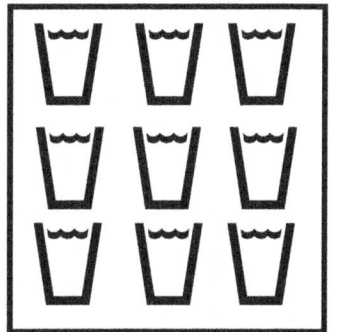

MEAL TRACKER

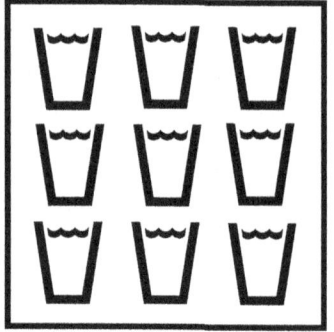

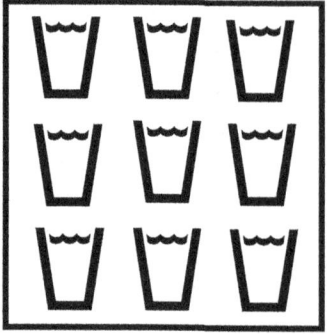

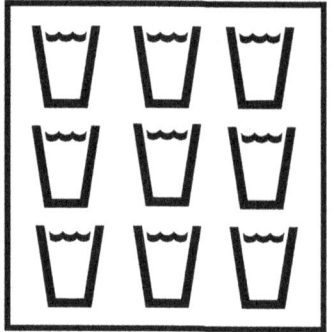

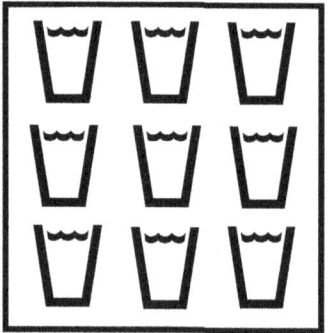

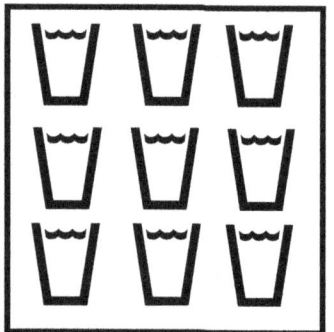

MEAL TRACKER

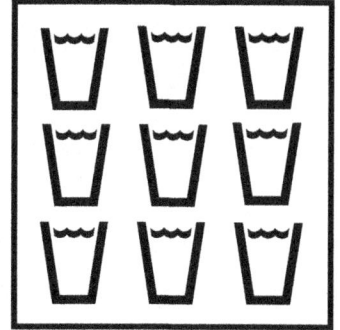

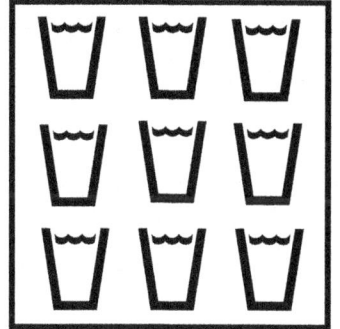

ROUND OVERVIEW

How many times did you eat fast food?

How many times did you cook your own meals?

Did you step out of your comfort zone with any meals?

How was your water intake?

What do you plan to change about your meals next round?

List 3 meals you'd like to cut out.

List 3 new meals you'd like to try.

ROUND OVERVIEW

DID YOU ACCOMPLISH YOUR GOAL WEIGHT? IF YES, WHAT DID YOU REWARD YOURSELF WITH AND WHY?

WERE YOU SUCCESSFUL IN CONTROLLING OR ENDING ANY BAD HABITS? WHICH HABITS DO YOU THINK WILL REQUIRE MORE OF YOUR TIME? DID YOU TAKE ON ANY GOOD HABITS? WHAT WERE THEY? WHAT HABITS ARE YOU INTERESTED IN WORKING ON NEXT ROUND?

HOW WERE YOUR MOODS THIS MONTH? WHAT HAVE YOU DONE FOR YOURSELF? HOW DO YOU FEEL AFTER COMPLETING THIS ROUND?

HOW'D THE SELF CARE REMINDER GO? HOW MANY TIMES DID YOU CATER TO YOURSELF? WHAT DO YOU HAVE PLANNED TO TREAT YOURSELF NEXT ROUND?

DID YOU TRY MEAL PLANNING THIS MONTH? DISCOVER ANY NEW RECIPES OR FOODS YOU ENJOYED? CHOOSE A DAY THAT WOULD BE GOOD FOR YOU TO MEAL PREP FOR THE WEEK.

HOW ACTIVE WERE YOU THIS ROUND? WHAT WAS YOUR MOST FREQUENT ACTIVITY? HOW DO YOU PLAN TO BE MORE ACTIVE NEXT ROUND? ANYTHING NEW YOU'D LIKE TO TRY?

WHAT DID YOUR SLEEP TRACKER REVEAL? HOW HAS IT CHANGED? TRY ANY OF OF THE TIPS/EXERCISES? WHICH ONES WERE HELPFUL?

ROUND 12

ENJOY THE JOURNEY.

Self-belief and hard
work will always earn
you success.
Virat Kohli

Goals

HABIT TRACKER

Here is where you'll track your habits. In this round the dates are provided so jot down the name of the habit you are working towards or determined to break on the line below. (Ex: Fast food, Exercise, Smoking, etc.) Each day you are successful in either achieving or breaking this habit, you'll highlight or circle the date. The ultimate goal as you continue on through your rounds is to have the whole month colored in. The key is to break bad habits and enforce good ones.

1 2 3 4 5 6 7 8 9
10 11 12 13 14 15 16
17 18 19 20 21 22 23
24 25 26 27 28 29
30 31

_____

1 2 3 4 5 6 7 8 9
10 11 12 13 14 15 16
17 18 19 20 21 22 23
24 25 26 27 28 29
30 31

_____

1 2 3 4 5 6 7 8 9
10 11 12 13 14 15 16
17 18 19 20 21 22 23
24 25 26 27 28 29
30 31

_____

1 2 3 4 5 6 7 8 9
10 11 12 13 14 15 16
17 18 19 20 21 22 23
24 25 26 27 28 29
30 31

_____

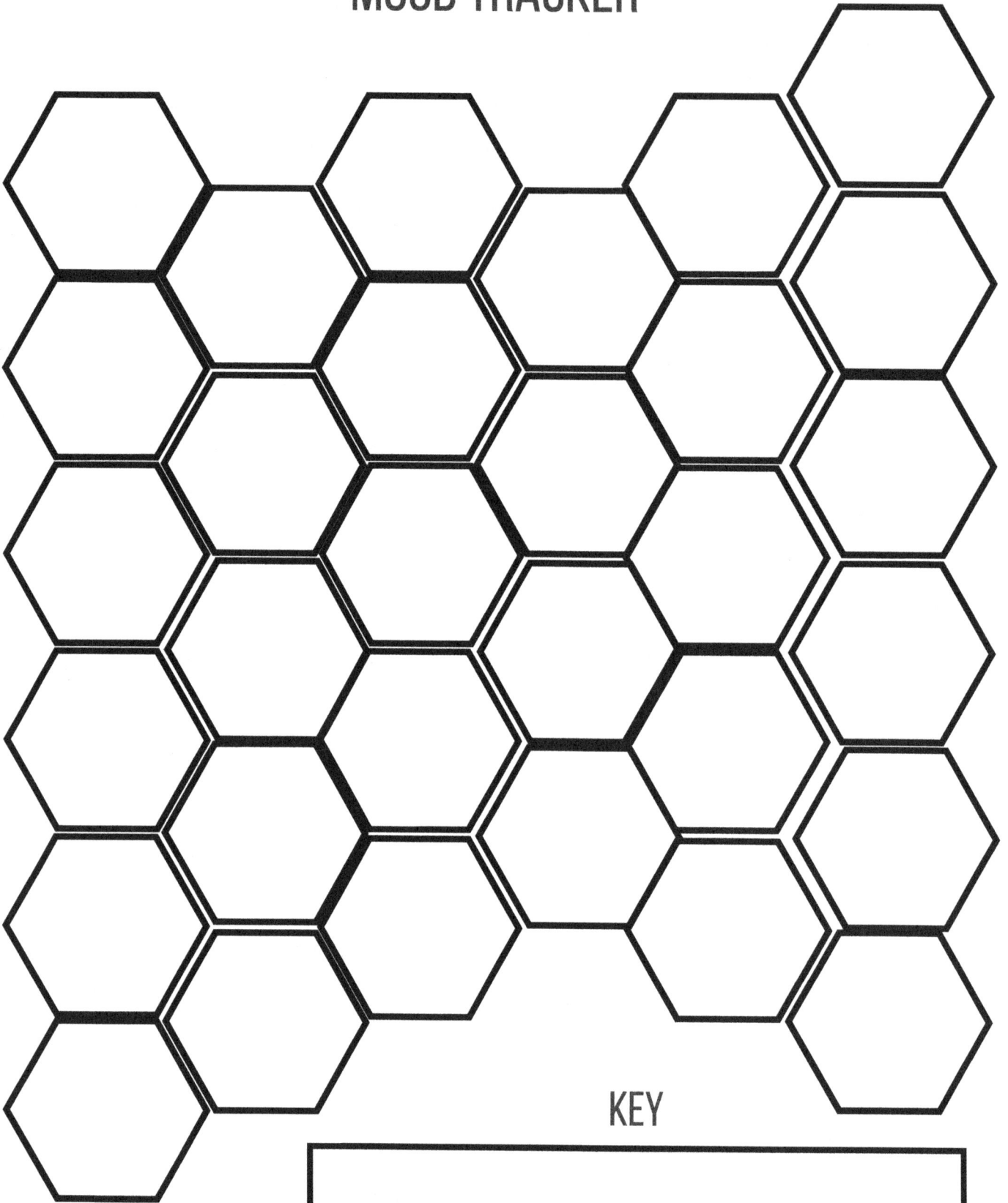

MOOD TRACKER

KEY

30 DAYS OF SELF CARE

For this portion you will list 30 acts of self care for each day this month. This is a challenge for you to spend a bit more time taking care of yourself. Be sure to include physical, mental and spiritual acts for the month. Cater to your overall health. When you've completed that task, come back and highlight it.

S	M	T	W	T	F	S

KEY

What Makes Me Happy?

This portion is a little different than the others. Here you will fill this page with ANY and EVERYTHING that makes you happy. This is a reflecting portion.

MENTAL HEALTH CHECK IN

This portion is a free write. Come back here as often as you'd like to pour out your feelings of how your journey is going. Some days are much harder than others and its helpful to get it out your head and jot it down. Just a few minutes a day, take a moment to free your mind here. You'll like to look back on this as well throughout your journey to reflect on your mindset at the start of your journey.

GRATITUDE LOG

This portion is a free write. Come back here as often as you'd like to pour out your feelings of gratitude during this round. You'll like to look back on this as well throughout your journey to reflect on your mindset at the start of your journey.

PROGRESS TRACKER

This portion is a mid journey reflection how how many pounds you've lost/gained so far on this journey & how much closer you are to your goal! List the date your journey began, as well as your starting weight and goal weight! Then draw circles or hearts in the bottom jar, representing how many pounds you've already lost/gained and do the same in the top jar representing how many more pounds are left to reach your goal weight for this journey!

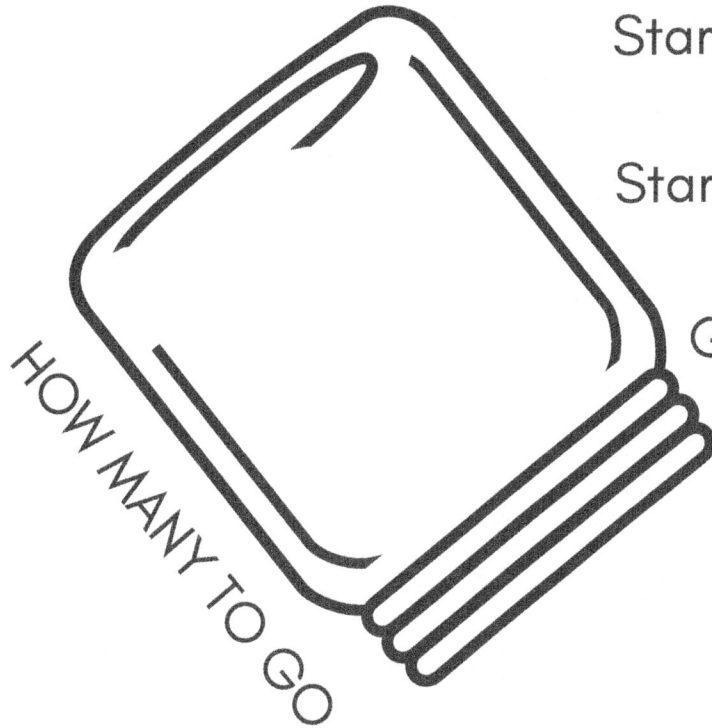

Start Date:

Starting Weight:

Goal Weight:

HOW MANY TO GO

LITTLE by LITTLE, a LITTLE becomes a **LOT**

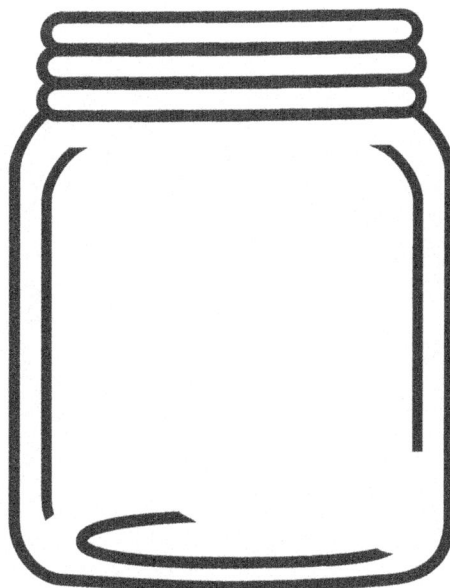

HOW MANY LOST/GAINED

SLEEP TRACKER

31
30
29
28
27
26
25
24
23
22
21
20
19
18
17
16
15
14
13
12
11
10
9
8
7
6
5
4
3
2
1

6 7 8 9 10 11 12 1 2 3 4 5 6 7 8 9 10 11 12

WORKOUT LOG

	S	M	T	W	T	F	S
WEEK 1							
WEEK 2							
WEEK 3							
WEEK 4							

KEY

MEAL TRACKER

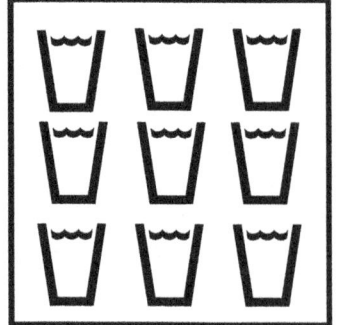

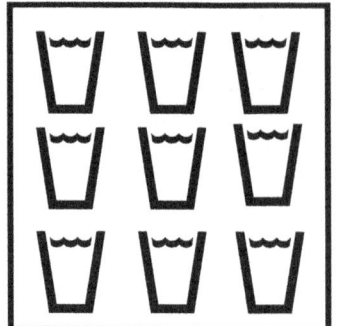

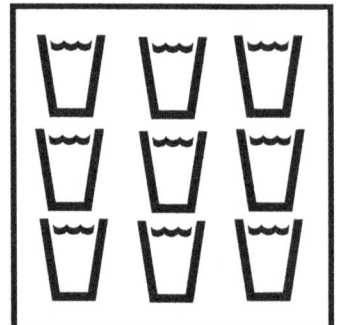

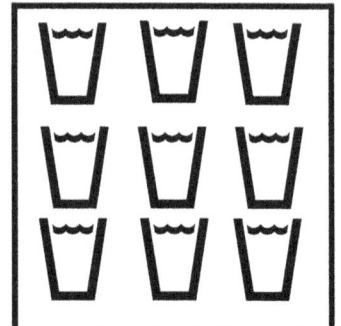

MEAL TRACKER

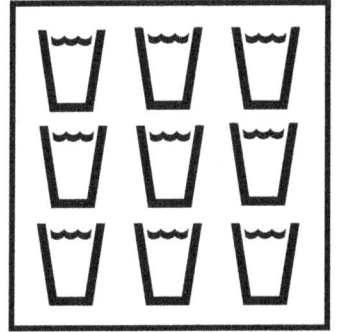

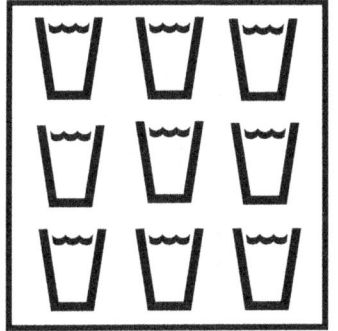

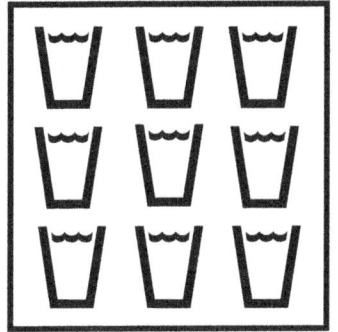

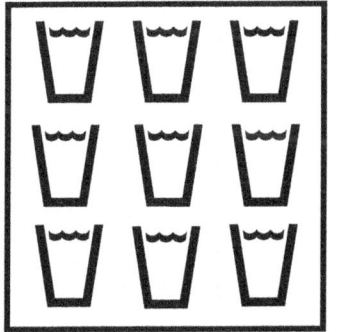

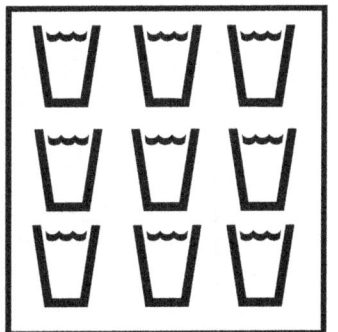

MEAL TRACKER

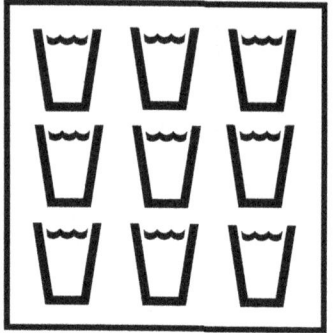

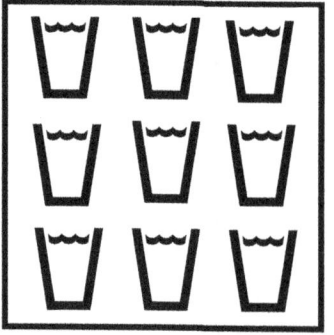

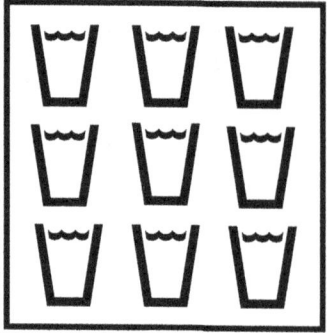

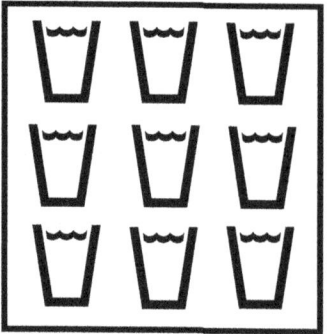

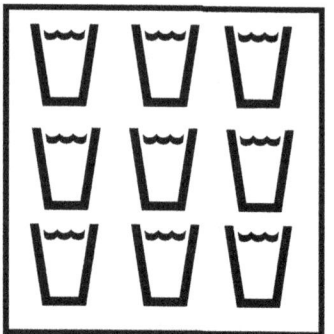

MEAL TRACKER

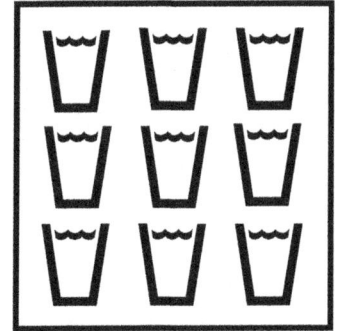

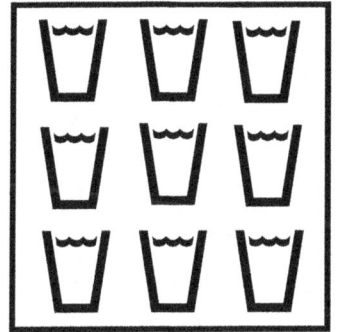

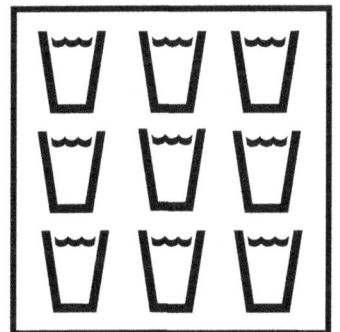

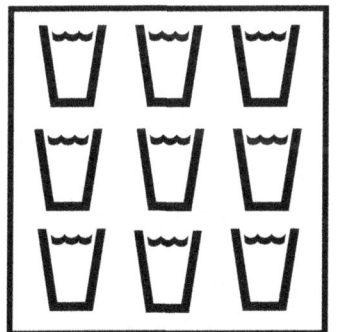

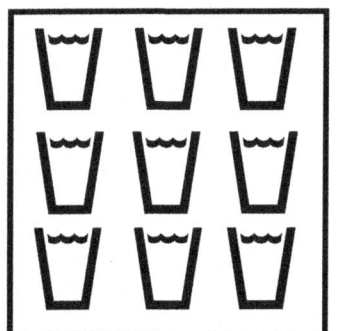

MEAL TRACKER

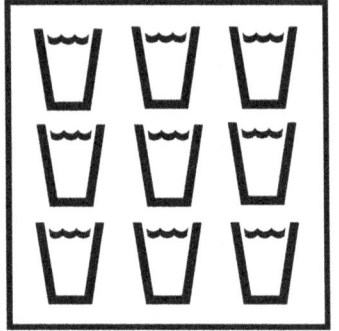

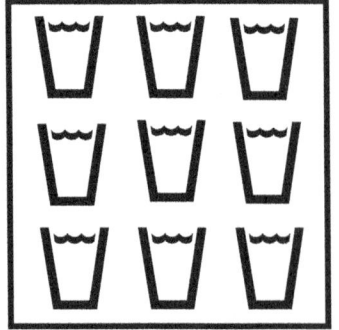

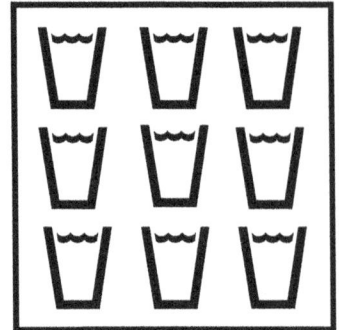

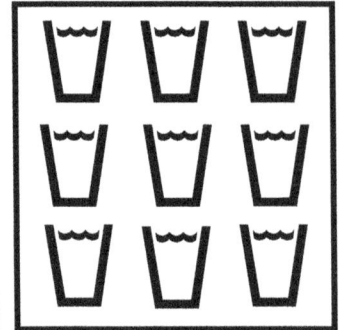

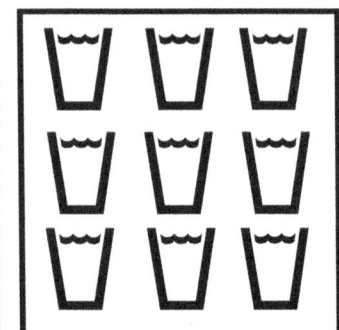

MEAL TRACKER

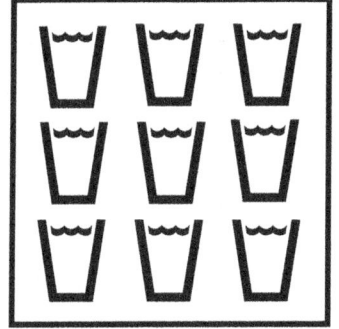

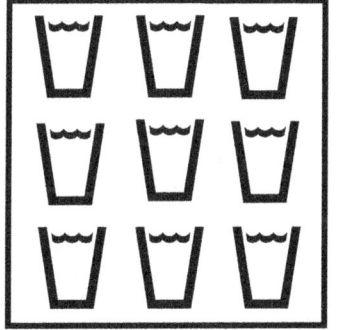

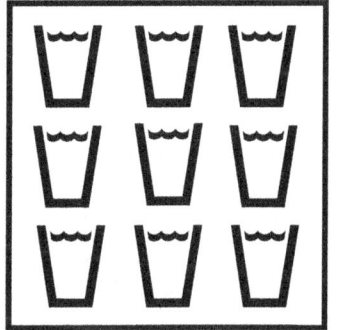

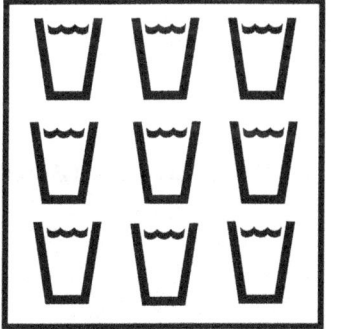

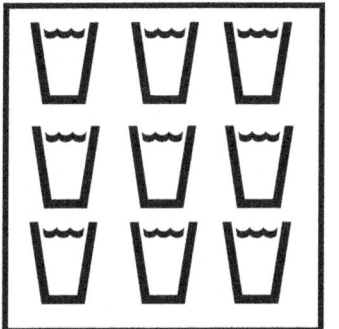

MEAL TRACKER

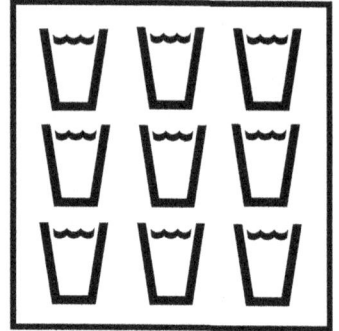

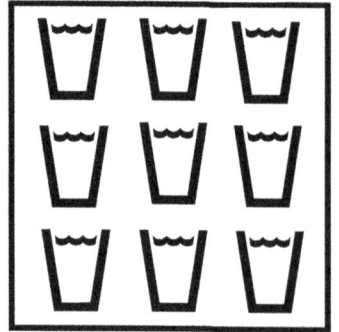

ROUND OVERVIEW

How many times did you eat fast food?

How many times did you cook your own meals?

Did you step out of your comfort zone with any meals?

How was your water intake?

List 3 meals you'd like to cut out.

List 3 new meals you'd like to try.

ROUND OVERVIEW

DID YOU ACCOMPLISH YOUR GOAL WEIGHT? IF YES, WHAT DID YOU REWARD YOURSELF WITH AND WHY? HOW DO YOU FEEL?

WERE YOU SUCCESSFUL IN CONTROLLING OR ENDING ANY BAD HABITS? WHICH HABITS DO YOU THINK WILL REQUIRE MORE OF YOUR TIME? DID YOU TAKE ON ANY GOOD HABITS? WHAT WERE THEY?

HOW WERE YOUR MOODS THIS MONTH? WHAT HAVE YOU DONE FOR YOURSELF? HOW DO YOU FEEL AFTER COMPLETING THIS ROUND?

HOW'D THE SELF CARE REMINDER GO? HOW MANY TIMES DID YOU CATER TO YOURSELF? WHAT DO YOU HAVE PLANNED TO TREAT YOURSELF FOR COMPLETING ALL 12 ROUNDS?

DID YOU MEAL PLAN AT ALL THIS MONTH? DISCOVER ANY NEW RECIPES OR FOODS YOU ENJOYED? WHEN IS YOUR MEAL PLANNING DAY?

HOW ACTIVE WERE YOU THIS ROUND? WHAT WAS YOUR MOST FREQUENT ACTIVITY? HOW MUCH MORE ACTIVE ARE YOU SINCE ROUND 1? ANYTHING NEW YOU'VE TRIED?

WHAT DID YOUR SLEEP TRACKER REVEAL? HOW HAS IT CHANGED? HOW HAS YOUR SLEEP IMPROVED THIS YEAR?

FINAL REFLECTIONS

WHAT GOALS ARE YOU MOST PROUD OF ACCOMPLISHING SINCE STARTING YOUR JOURNEY?

REFLECTING ON BAD HABITS FROM ROUND 1, WHAT HABITS HAVE YOU ELIMINATED AND GAINED DURING THIS JOURNEY?

HOW HAVE YOUR MOODS BEEN OVER THE LAST 12 ROUNDS? DO YOU NOTICE IMPROVEMENTS? HAVE YOU BEEN DOING MORE ACTIVITIES & SPENDING TIME WITH THOSE WHO BRING YOU HAPPINESS?

HOW HELPFUL HAS THE MENTAL CHECK IN BEEN? DO YOU LOG FREQUENTLY?

HOW HELPFUL HAS THE GRATITUDE LOG BEEN? DO YOU LOG FREQUENTLY?

FINAL REFLECTIONS

IF YOU'RE READING THIS, YOU'VE COMPLETED 12 ROUNDS! YOU DID IT! WHILE YOU HAVE FINISHED THIS JOURNAL, THE JOURNEY NEVER ENDS. WHAT VALUABLE LESSONS HAVE YOU LEARNED ABOUT YOURSELF ON THIS JOURNEY? WHAT WILL YOU IMPLEMENT AS YOU CONTINUE THIS JOURNEY OF SELF LOVE AND DISCOVERY?

HOW HAS YOUR SELF CONFIDENCE IMPROVED SINCE STARTING THIS JOURNEY? HOW HAVE YOU STEPPED OUT OF YOUR COMFORT ZONE SINCE ROUND 1?

HOW HELPFUL HAS YOUR MANTRA BEEN? DO YOU RECITE IT DAILY? DO YOU HAVE IT MEMORIZED YET?

LIST A FEW WORDS OF ENCOURAGEMENT FOR YOURSELF DURING THE REMAINDER OF YOUR JOURNEY.

GETTING TO KNOW YOU

This portion is for reflection. You've completed the 12 rounds, so take a look at all your "Getting To Know You" entries and express the obstacles you've overcame and who you are today. Share the lessons you've learned about yourself and how you stayed motivated throughout this journey. How has this journal helped you on your journey? Have you achieved all your goals? How is your mental space? How do you plan to celebrate this accomplishment?

RESULTS

This is reflection portion. Share a photo of you at the beginning of this journey and a photo of you now. Tape or glue the photos side by side and date them if you can. Be proud of your growth. You have accomplished a great deal and should reward yourself!

MANTRA

When you embarked on this journey a year ago, you wrote a mantra for yourself that helped you along this journey. Now, a year later, take a look at that mantra and use this portion to write yourself a new one. It can be as long or as short as you like, but remember you will start each day repeating this to yourself and eventually will memorize it. Use positive words such as "I will", "When I", I can", I am", etc. Speak all you want to achieve now and beyond this journey into existence.. Don't overthink. Just express freely.

FINAL THOUGHTS

This portion is a free write. Jot down your feelings about this journey and your goals to come. I am so proud of you for committing to this and joining me on this journey! The journey continues on and I hope this journal has provided you with the necessary tools needed to keep on fighting those obstacles and encouraged you to allow yourself all the room you need to grow. I hope that you love yourself more now than you did on Day one. I hope you trust yourself more. I hope this journal has brought you peace. Congratulations for completing this yearlong journey and good luck to you on your future endeavors!

Made in the USA
Monee, IL
19 June 2020